THE MEDICAL PROFESSION IN INDIA

THE MEDICAL PROFESSION IN INDIA

PATRICK HEHIR

GYAN

Published by

GYAN

Gyan Publishing House
5, Ansari Road
Daryaganj, New Delhi-110002
Phone: 011-47034999, 9811692060
E-mail: books@gyanbooks.com

Distribution Network
gyanbooks.com
India, USA, Canada, UK, Australia

ISBN: 978-93-6780-402-5 (HB)

First Published, 1923

2nd Impression 2024

Printed at: Gyan Press, Delhi.

THE MEDICAL PROFESSION IN INDIA
Author: PATRICK HEHIR

THE MEDICAL PROFESSION IN INDIA

OXFORD MEDICAL PUBLICATIONS

THE MEDICAL PROFESSION IN INDIA

BY

MAJOR-GENERAL SIR PATRICK HEHIR
K.C.I.E., C.B., C.M.G., I.M.S.

LONDON
HENRY FROWDE AND HODDER & STOUGHTON
THE *LANCET* BUILDING
1 BEDFORD STREET, STRAND, W.C.2

CONTENTS

THE MEDICAL PROFESSION IN INDIA

INTRODUCTION

WESTERN medicine in India is at present going through a critical stage of its history, one that is likely seriously to affect its development and advancement. This crisis has arisen from many causes, among which the chief are the following: The Indian Medical Service has lost its attraction for young graduates of the home medical schools, because of the rapid Indianization of that service following the Reforms Scheme, leading to uncertainty regarding the future and to the filling of the professorial chairs of the medical colleges and college hospitals, and many of the higher civil medical appointments, with Indians; the shortage of medical men in the United Kingdom which enables those who a few years ago would have formed the I.M.S. to seek and readily obtain employment at home; and the great fillip that has been given to the ancient systems of medicine. The general effect is one of retrogression, and if a decidedly radical change is not instituted at an early date, there is little risk in prophesying a decline in the efficiency and skill with which orthodox medicine and surgery will be practised in our Indian Empire in the future.

The provincial legislatives convey the impression that the demise of the I.M.S. would not in any way disturb their peace of mind; indeed, one province has declared that it does not want the services of any I.M.S. officers. Those who know what a calamity to India the disappearance of the Europeans of the I.M.S. would be, view with no small degree of surprise the supineness of the authorities who have it in their power to prevent it, and hope ardently that the real situation will be appreciated before it is too late.

Ever since the middle of the eighteenth century Western medicine has been fighting against prejudices, apathy, and ancient systems of treatment, which to-day present more formidable resistance than modern science is prepared to encounter. Many will agree with me that this long contest, which until lately was waged successfully, should not be abandoned without making a final struggle.

I have spent the greater part of my life in India, and have had a wide experience in filling almost every sort of appointment in military life, and many in civil life, including that of lecturer on various subjects, health officer of a large municipality for ten years, general practitioner, and consulting physician. I have contributed for thirty-five years to Indian medical periodicals on questions of the day, and been a member of many committees connected with the organization of the medical services in India, Indian station hospitals, etc., and I may claim to have some degree of familiarity with medical work in India. I began my medical education as a student in the Medical College of Calcutta. I had a happy, interesting, and, some have been generous enough to say, a somewhat useful life in that country. It is a subject for regret to many, who like myself have given the best years of their life to service in India, to observe the falling off that is now in progress, and which has impelled me to place the facts before the medical profession of the Empire.

To enable us to understand fully the present position and form an opinion as to how the set-back which Western medicine has had may be met, it is necessary to consider the composition of the medical profession in India, including the various Government services; medical education with its advantages and shortcomings; the independent medical profession; public health work; and the ancient systems of medicine practised.

Composition of the Medical Profession in India

There is no country in the world in which the medical profession is more heterogeneously represented than in India. Medical and surgical treatment is carried out by persons who range from the most highly qualified and competent exponents of Western methods to mystics who adopt the Ayurvedic and Unani systems, but know little or nothing about them. For convenience, however, it may be stated that the profession in India consists of three groups—the medical services of Government, independent medical practitioners, and those who practise the ancient systems.

1. *The medical services of Government.*—These include those employed with the Army in India, and those in civil employ. In the Army we have R.A.M.C. officers and military assistant surgeons who look after British troops, and officers of the I.M.S. and military sub-assistant surgeons who look after Indian troops. These are all under the Director of Medical Services in India, who has hitherto always been an officer of the Army Medical Service; he is the adviser of the Commander-in-Chief in India on medical and sanitary matters. The A.M.S. also hold ten administrative appointments with commands and districts; a corresponding number of administrative posts are held by I.M.S. officers.

On the civil side, the Director-General, Indian Medical Service, who is the Surgeon-General with the Imperial Government, is the head administrative officer; the other administrative officers are the Surgeon-General with the Bengal, Bombay, and Madras Governments, and the Inspectors-General of Civil Hospitals, one with each local government, all of the I.M.S.; civil surgeons, made up of I.M.S. officers (lent to local governments), civil and military and assistant surgeons, and civil and military sub-assistant surgeons. At each district headquarters there is a civil surgeon who has under him a civil assistant surgeon, and one or more civil sub-assistant surgeons;

all officers now employed by local governments, except those of the I.M.S., are entirely provincial. A number of Europeans and Indians hold specialist appointments, such as bacteriologists or analytical chemists. The duties discharged by the Government medical services include, on the military side, administrative and executive medical and sanitary work of the whole Army in India; on the civil side, administrative and executive work of all State hospitals and dispensaries, medical treatment of all Government servants, medico-legal work of the country, medical and sanitary work of jails, lunatic and leper asylums, sanitation of the Indian Empire and medical education. The duties carried out by the officers of the I.M.S. are probably among the most important functions of any department in India; there is little doubt that the medical services of the State exercise a certain amount of political influence for good which is dependent on the close relation which medical duties establish in the population as a whole. As the Government medical services—especially the civil—form the backbone of the medical work done in India, they will be referred to more in detail later on.

2. *The independent medical profession.*—This is mainly made up of graduates and licentiates of the universities of India, diplomates of the official and unofficial medical schools, retired civil and military assistant surgeons and sub-assistant surgeons, failed students of the medical colleges and schools, and a host of unqualified persons who practise allopathic medicine. There are also many Indians who have British degrees or diplomas, men who went through the whole or part of their curriculum in the U.K.; and many Europeans who either practise independently or are employed by various companies in tea gardens, factories, and on railways. There are now also a fair number of Indian women practising Western medicine, some in independent practice, others in the Women's Medical Service under the Central Committee of the Dufferin Fund, whilst a good few are being employed by

municipalities and district boards for work in local hospitals; the same may be said of a number of European lady doctors who qualified at home or in India and are similarly employed.

Homœopathy is practised by a certain number, some of whom obtained qualification after examinations in scientific medicine, but most of whom are unqualified.

3. *The practitioners of Ayurvedic and Unani systems.*—These, collectively, greatly outnumber those who practise Western medicine; no census has been taken, and so far registration has not been made compulsory; many thousands of quacks practise these systems, who, whilst they do some good, also do much harm. These references to charlatanism ought not to create surprise. We had our quacks in the U.K. for centuries, and it was not until the Registration Act of 1858 was brought into operation that any serious hindrance was placed in their way; India is going through the same experience now with her Medical Registration Act of 1916. Quackery in India is still widespread, and it is very desirable to extend registration to all who are eligible for it and are practising Western medicine.

Nurses.—A large number of highly qualified nursing sisters are employed in Government and other hospitals, who are chiefly to supervise, guide, and instruct the subordinate nursing staff in these institutions, or are connected with certain corporate bodies such as the Lady Minto Nursing Association, which provides nursing sisters for Europeans in India, while some practise independently. Many well-qualified and registered midwives are also employed in Government and private hospitals, and some of them practise independently; but there are many thousands of unqualified indigenous midwives or *dhais* who are ignorant, uneducated, unclean in their habits, carry on their work unsupervised, and are responsible for many deaths and an enormous amount of suffering—"dirty midwifery" is responsible for thousands of deaths annually and untold suffering.

CHAPTER I

MEDICAL EDUCATION IN INDIA

MEDICAL education in India is carried out in the medical colleges and college hospitals connected with the various universities and in various medical schools and their hospitals. The universities grant to successful *alumni* degrees which are registrable in the U.K. and in India, and licences to practise, which, though registrable in India, are, so far, not registrable in the U.K. The General Medical Council of Great Britain has lately threatened to withdraw the privilege of registration in England because of insufficient training in midwifery of graduates and licentiates of Indian universities; this is dealt with more in detail later on. There are also a few unofficial medical colleges and medical schools unconnected with the universities and uncontrolled by Government, which award licences to practise; these qualifications are not registrable in the U.K., nor in India, and during the last generation or so a great evil has sprung up through medical diplomas being granted by unauthorized bodies.

Medical schools exist in various parts of the country; in these the standard is lower, the curriculum less elaborate, and the duration of training shorter than in the colleges; successful students are granted a State diploma to practise which, until recently, was not registrable (*vide infra*).

All the official medical colleges and hospitals connected with them aim at giving a medical education equal to that obtainable in the corresponding institutions of the U.K.; to what extent they succeed in this is referred to later on; it should be remembered that medical colleges were not started until about seventy or eighty years ago, that until fifty years or so ago the preliminary education of the youths of India was not sufficiently high to enable them to assimilate medical scientific subjects successfully. An Indian who has been educated up to the matriculation standard is not able to absorb the teaching in medical and scientific subjects in the same way as a European similarly educated—he has not the same working knowledge of English. When lecturing to matriculation lads I found it necessary to talk in the simplest language possible, not always an easy task in technical subjects.

Medical education in India, like the independent medical profession, is still in an undeveloped state. It is not at present possible for a medical student to get a complete medical education; not one of the universities is fully prepared either in staff or equipment to give the medical education that can be obtained in our home universities. No one is to blame for this; it is simply a question of evolution; the history of medicine in India shows this distinctly.

Western medical education began in India just a century ago by the creation of what was called a "school for native doctors" in Calcutta, in 1822. Let us briefly review the history of medical education in the Presidencies; I take that of Bengal, with which I am familiar; this history will show what an up-hill task allopathic medicine had in establishing itself in the country. After the school for native doctors had been running for some years a committee appointed by Government reported that the school was very defective owing to the absence of a proper qualifying preliminary education, the omission of the practical teaching of anatomy, shortness of the periods of study, and for other reasons. Medical education in the Ayurvedic and Unani systems was being carried out separately in the Sanskrit College of Calcutta under Dr. Madhusudan Gupta (*vide infra*) and Unani medicine in the Madrassah (Mahomedan) College also in Calcutta. In January 1835 the school for native doctors and the medical classes on the Ayurvedic and Unani systems were abolished, and the Calcutta Medical College opened. The teaching was in English; there were fifty foundation pupils receiving a stipend, who were to spend from four to six years at the College and to be required to learn the principles and practice of medical science in strict accordance with the mode adopted in Europe. . . . In addition to the pupils on the foundation, the benefits of the College were to be thrown open to all classes of native youths between 14 and 20 without distinction of class or creed, if they fulfilled certain conditions. The Superintendent of the College, with the aid of an assistant, was expected to instruct these latter pupils in anatomy, medicine, and midwifery, and to qualify them for medical charges, civil and military.[1] Dr. Madhusudan Gupta was transferred to the new institution and had two assistants assigned to him. From 1837 to 1856 the Medical College was administered by a council with a secretary, then the government of the College was handed over to a council formed by the professors with the principal as president. At first there was no hospital attached to the College; the students had to attend a few small hospitals in the city for clinical work. In 1838 a small hospital was connected with the College, then a larger one, and finally in 1852–53 the present College Hospital was erected, the professors of the College becoming its physicians and surgeons. In 1839 the vernacular classes were recommenced. In the same year European and Armenian students were admitted to the College. Up to 1845 the course was four years. In 1846 the London University, the R.C.P., and the Society of Apothecaries of London recognized the College curriculum. In the following year a two-years' course (which was later extended to three years) was instituted for "hospital apprentices" (descendants of Europeans and Eurasians occupying subordinate positions), who became on qualifying a subordinate medical service for duty with British troops; they were the predecessors of the Military Assistant Surgeon branch of the present Indian Medical Depart-

[1] *Report of the Calcutta Univ. Com.*, Part I, chap. xxiii.

ment. In 1851–52 a Bengali vernacular class was organized in the College. In 1860 the medical examinations of the College were handed over to the University of Calcutta, which granted a licence in medicine and surgery (L.M.S.) to successful matriculates, and M.B. to first arts *alumni*. Other degrees were added. At this time it will be seen there were four classes in the Medical College :

1. Primary, who went through the full university curriculum of five years ; and

2. Three classes each pursuing a three-year course, viz. (*a*) Hospital Apprentice class, (*b*) Hindustani Class, and (*c*) Bengali Class. The curriculum of 2 (*b*) and (*c*) was the same, and the diploma of L.M.S. was conferred on successful candidates at the end of the course, which did not include midwifery.

In 1864 the Bengali Class was divided into a Higher and Lower. The Higher students were educated in minor medicine and surgery and became private practitioners to the poorer classes ; the Lower were similarly educated to fill certain posts in Government service ; both received a vernacular licentiateship in medicine and surgery. In 1868 midwifery, diseases of women and children, chemistry, and medical jurisprudence were added to their subjects.

The Medical College gradually became overcrowded. In 1873 the two vernacular classes had 823 pupils, and had to be transferred to another newly created institution, the Campbell Medical School in Sealdah (a near suburb of Calcutta), which was connected with a large municipal hospital taken over by Government. The Hindustani classes were discontinued. In 1874 the Dacca and Patna Medical Schools were opened and connected with good hospitals, and later a medical school was opened at Cuttack.

To continue with the Medical College of Calcutta. After some years the prerequisite for entrants for university qualifications was raised to the first arts examination. "For many years the university granted two qualifications to first arts pupils at the end of an undergraduate course of five years—L.M.S. and M.B. At that time the students entered for both qualifications, the M.B. being an honours degree compared with the L.M.S., but the large majority only succeeded in obtaining the licence; thus, in 1901–2, sixty-four took the latter and only two the M.B. In 1906 the L.M.S. was to be removed from the list of university qualifications after a certain number of years (the last L.M.S. examination was held in 1913) and the course was extended to six years; the matriculation was again introduced and substituted for the F.A. as an entrance qualification of the course, and, in addition to the higher degree of M.D., there were instituted the degrees of M.S., M.D., and D.P.H."[1]

The regulations of the Calcutta University M.B. are formed on the general lines of those of the corresponding degree of the London University, but differ somewhat in detail. The majority of the present *alumni* have passed the first arts or first B.Sc., but there are also many B.A.s and B.Sc.s. Students entering as matriculates generally fail to pass the examinations and thus block the way for others, as they must go through the courses of the subjects in which they fail before being eligible for re-examination.

As previously shown, the teaching in the Calcutta Medical College was initially very elementary. The first course of lectures and demonstrations on anatomy was given on clay models, samples of which are still to be seen in the Calcutta Museum. Before the advent of the British Raj the rational treatment of disease did not exist in the country. When the H.E.I.C. took over the Dewani Administration of Bengal only the rich could avail themselves of medical treatment by the European doctors who were employed under the Company; the middle and poorer classes of Indians were left to the tender mercies of charlatans, bonesetters, *hakims*, and *vaids*. From an early stage of our occupation Western medicine was appreciated by many Indians, but they could not avail themselves of it for want of dispensaries and hospitals. In Calcutta at first one charitable dispensary was opened,

[1] *Report of the Calcutta Univ. Com.* Part 1, chap. xxiii.

and later, in 1792, a small civil hospital. One of the earliest questions considered by us was the medical education of Indian youths, but apathy combined with superstition prevented anything of importance being done until 1835, when the Viceroy, Lord William Bentinck, opened the Calcutta Medical College: at first there was great difficulty in finding sufficient students of the educated classes. Tempting facilities were offered, but the Brahmin youths and other higher Hindu castes would not join; they specially objected to anatomy classes and dissections, touching dead bodies, and handling the sick of the lower castes, although both the *Sushruta Samhita* and the Shastras show beyond all doubt that anatomical dissection was adopted by Hindus two thousand years ago; modern custom, however, prevailed. Eventually, under the fostering care of the Council of Medical Education, the lower-class Sudras were replaced by Brahmins, Kyasthras, and Baidas. The 10th January 1836 was the most memorable day in the annals of Western medicine in India; the late Pundit Madhusudan Gupta (already referred to) entered the dissecting-room of the Calcutta Medical College and touched a dead body and became the first demonstrator of anatomy in the College. I recall with much pleasure many conversations I had with this venerable and distinguished reformer, whose bust now adorns the College. The better classes of Indians fully recognized the importance of this incident, which was celebrated by a public holiday, illuminations, and universal exultation.

The present Medical College Hospital is built on the old block principle, and periodically its wards used to get highly infected. I can personally remember the days when charcoal in wire net baskets suspended from the ceilings was used to purify the air of the wards; whole wards were at times vacated an account of either hospital gangrene or sepsis, and I was told by my lamented and talented friend the late Lieut.-Col. Edward Lawrie, I.M.S., of a time when one of the surgical wards was kept vacant for weeks after an epidemic of tetanus in it. In the early days of the hospital the nursing was very primitive; the house surgeons and house physicians were responsible for the feeding, and in important cases the food was given by students on duty.

The Medical Hospital and its annexes have at present accommodation for patients and clinical teaching as follows:

The Hospital itself: 320 beds for medical and surgical cases;

Prince of Wales Hospital: 88 beds for aseptic surgery;

Eden Hospital: 105 gynecological cases;

Eye Infirmary: 51 beds;

Paying patients' block: 12 beds;

Cholera ward: 20 beds;

Ezra Hospital: 20 beds for Jewish patients.

Total 616 beds.

Connected with the hospital is a large training school for nurses and a class for native midwives (*dhais*).

At present two classes of students are admitted into the Calcutta Medical College:

(1) *Regular students*, male and female, the majority of whom go through the university course; a small number do the course for the State Medical Faculty examination (*vide infra*).

(2) *Military students*, who go through a special course to meet the requirements of the military authorities; they become, on passing the prescribed examination, military assistant surgeons.

There is a limited number of *casual students* who take special classes; these are usually men who come to the U.K. to graduate in one of our universities.

The final selection of candidates of class (1) to enter the College rests with the Principal, and of class (2) with the Director-General, Indian Medical Service. Of class (1) a certain number of vacancies are reserved for students from the adjacent provinces. The number of university pupils admitted each year is usually 120, which may be increased to 150. The number of candidates is always vastly in excess of the vacancies. In 1918–19 there were

887 applications for 142 vacancies. Of the female students the majority are Hindus. When I visited the College in March 1919 there were seventeen women pupils; they must live in a hostel which is near the College; they get their medical education free.

The arrangements for teaching general medicine and surgery are excellent; the dissecting-room, physiological and pathological laboratories are as good as are to be met with in most of our home universities. The facilities for teaching the medical preliminary subjects, such as biology, physics, and chemistry, are not altogether satisfactory; personally I entertain serious doubts as to whether a medical college is quite the best place for tuition in these science subjects.

There are a few private medical colleges and schools in the country; these are practically all confined to Bengal. The Belgachia Medical College near Calcutta was the first non-official medical college managed and staffed entirely by Indians; it was started by Indian medical practitioners in 1886; it is connected with the Albert Victor Hospital of 200 beds. It has been amalgamated with another non-official institution, the College of Physicians and Surgeons of Bengal, which was started in 1897–8. There has for years been great pressure for admission to this combined college, and only a fraction of the applicants can gain entrance.

In 1915 the Government promised to make a capital grant of five lakhs of rupees for buildings, and an annual grant of Rs. 50,000 to this combined institution on the conditions that the College erected and fitted up the necessary laboratories and the required equipment, got affiliated to the Calcutta University, sent its pupils up for the University examinations, raised 2½ lakhs of rupees initially, and secured an annual grant of Rs. 30,000 from the Calcutta Corporation, meeting the remainder of the recurring cost from fees and endowments. Government was to nominate three members on a managing committee of eleven, and the appointment of the Superintendent of the hospital was to be subject to their approval. These conditions were, I understood, accepted and so far have been complied with. The College was formally opened in 1916 and affiliated to the Calcutta University up to the first M.B. examination. When I was in Calcutta in 1919 the number of pupils in the College was 275. Because of the paucity of hospital accommodation for patients and the limited facilities for clinical teaching and for other reasons the Calcutta University declined to grant affiliation for the other examinations for the M.B. degree. I was informed that more extended hospital accommodation was being arranged for, and more complete equipment for teaching the senior subjects was being acquired, and that when this task was carried out affiliation to the University for the full M.B. examinations was to be granted.

Several other teaching medical institutions were opened in Calcutta early in this century, but they are now defunct. Another, the National Medical School, has just been started.

In general terms it may be stated that a somewhat similar history holds good regarding the introduction and progress of Western medical education and medical work in the Madras and Bombay Presidencies.

Nothing has been done so far as regards the creation of non-Government medical colleges in Bombay and Madras ; there is no reason whatever, except want of local enterprise on the part of the independent medical profession and the wealthy part of the Indian public, why large and useful medical colleges should not be erected and worked in Bombay, Madras, and several of the large provincial towns and connected with their universities.

All the medical colleges in India, except the combined one above referred to, are Imperial ; their medical staffs are Government officers ; the postings of professors to the colleges are theoretically Imperial, but to a very large extent in practice provincial. Vacancies are filled up by the governors of the provinces with the sanction of the Imperial Government—such sanction is rarely refused.

If there is no suitable candidate on the provincial list the Imperial Government is requisitioned for a man. The Provincial Government asks its administrative medical officer regarding a candidate, he consults the principal of the college concerned, who consults his professional staff, and a man is selected.

All local governments have one or more *medical schools* under them, and regulate the admissions and training of the students taught in these institutions. The term *medical school* in India is applied to institutions in which the standard of medical education is lower than that given in the medical colleges which educate for university degrees and licentiateships. The control and management are vested in the superintendent of the school (who is a selected senior officer of the I.M.S.), under the supervision of the Surgeon-General or Inspector-General of civil hospitals of the province. Under the Bengal Government, for instance, there are the Campbell Medical School of Calcutta and the Medical School at Dacca, to which has just been added the Ronaldshay Medical School at Burdwan; under the Bihar and Orissa Government we have the medical schools at Patna and Cuttack; under the United Provinces Government is the Agra Medical School, and so on. Practically all the medical schools now require entrants to be over 16, and to have obtained a preliminary educational certificate equivalent to that of a university matriculation; students have to go through a four-years' medical curriculum; all teaching has to be in English. The pupils on complying with all the conditions of the school, and passing the examinations, obtain a licence to practise medicine. In 1914 a State Medical Faculty of Bengal was established for examining the students of the Bengal and other Medical Schools which might be recognized for the purpose by the Bengal Council of Medical Registration. The successful students become Licentiates of the State Medical Faculty of Bengal, a qualification which is registrable under the Bengal Medical Act of 1914. This Act established the first Medical Registration Council in India and a Medical Registrar for the Province of Bengal. Similar Acts have been introduced into all the local provinces (see sections on military assistant surgeons and civil sub-assistant surgeons).

A very large number of students are trained in these various medical schools annually; *e.g.* in 1919, the Campbell Medical School had 500 under training, the Dacca Medical School 400, and Agra 800. In these schools women are accepted who produce certificates of having passed the Middle School Scholarship examination (or other higher preliminary educational test), have a certificate of good character and are over 17; various scholarships are awarded to both male and female entrants.

There is a great demand for additional *medical schools* for the education of men of lower medical attainments, men of the old native-doctor class whose requirements in life can be met with greatly-reduced fees for work in rural districts. How to meet this demand has not yet been satisfactorily solved. Many thousands of medical men of this type are required in the districts and away from the large towns. That wise statesman Dr. M. N. Banerjee proposed in the Imperial Legislative Council in 1916 the following very important resolution which was accepted by Government: "That this Council recommends to the G.-G. in C. that local governments be asked to consider the advisability of establishing institutions for the purpose of giving medical students a special training conducted in the vernaculars so as to qualify them for ordinary medical practitioners in rural areas, and of encouraging and assisting deserving private enterprise to provide such medical education." To this all Anglo-Indians would give cordial approval, although many of us might consider the use of the vernacular instead of English retrograde, for the fundamental reason that there are few textbooks in vernacular, and of those in existence fewer still are up-to-date. Sir Pardey Lukis was in favour of this motion with the modification that the standard of medical education required for medical men in rural areas should be something of the kind that was given to the native doctors (already referred to) when Western medical education was first commenced in India. Lord Ronaldshay, Governor of Bengal, as one of his last official functions opened the Medical School at Burdwan mentioned above, which has been called after him. It is training men to a standard equal to that of the civil sub-assistant surgeon class. I would take the liberty of saying that on the occasion under reference Lord Ronaldshay expressed what many experienced medical men who have spent the best part of their lives in India consider should be the policy of all provincial governments in regard to any additional *medical schools* opened. He said : " The policy of the Government of Bengal had for some years been to establish at different centres of the province medical schools designed to provide a steady output of men with a sound though not unduly ambitious training in medicine on up-to-date Western lines ; in other words to turn out a general practitioner whose knowledge will be sufficiently high and whose fees will be sufficiently low to prove of practical benefit to the vast population of moderate means which inhabits the villages of Bengal. . . . The more urgent need at the present time is a large increase of a type of doctor corresponding to the country doctor in England, and it is the provision of this type that is aimed at in the establishment of this School." [1] The School was opened on January 16, 1922. It was scarcely opened when there were eight applicants for every vacancy available. There is an excellent hospital connected with the School. All such institutions are, of course, of little use without having attached to them hospitals for clinical teaching.

Another medical college is to be opened in Calcutta, the National Medical College. On July 8, 1922, Sir Surendra Nath Banerjee, Minister of Public Health, Bengal Government, presided over the inaugural meeting in connexion with this College. It is to work in association with King's Hospital and be affiliated to the State Medical Faculty.

[1] *The Pioneer Mail*, January 20, 1922.

2

Sir Surendra Nath Banerjee said that " reference had been made to the paucity of qualified medical practitioners in India. He, on behalf of the Bengal Government, assured the meeting that the Government would rejoice if more medical schools were established. He announced that two more medical schools were likely to be shortly established, one in connexion with Sambunath Pandit Hospital, and another at Howrah. They were going to start some more medical schools in the mofussil; one at Myminsingh, and in the course of a year medical schools would be started at Chittagong and Berhampore. He appealed to the landed aristocracy to co-operate with the Government in saving human lives and mitigating human suffering."[1] This is most satisfactory; Bengal is far ahead of any other province in the matter of increasing the number of its medical schools for the class of men that are most urgently wanted for work in rural areas, and it is earnestly hoped that other provinces will follow this excellent example.

The few Government medical colleges and schools in existence can give tuition to a very small proportion of those who seek admission within their portals; and it is not possible for the Imperial or local governments to continue to develop and increase the number of unofficial medical colleges and medical schools. One hopes that the day is not remote when there will be several unofficial medical colleges and schools officered entirely by Indians of the independent profession; and that these institutions will be affiliated to the various universities (initially at least), connected with large non-Government hospitals supported by voluntary subscription, and that they will be found working side by side with the corresponding official institutions in friendly competition. " Let them (the independent medical profession) unite and found medical colleges of their own "; this was the advice of one of the wisest Directors-General the I.M.S. has ever produced—the late Lieut.-Gen. Sir Pardey Lukis. It is

[1] *The Pioneer Mail*, July 14, 1922.

up to the wealthy public of India to create unofficial medical colleges and college hospitals with entirely Indian staffs in many centres in India; this will be the most laudable manner in which their wealth can be spent for the benefit of the whole population, and especially for the relief of the poor; it would, incidentally, greatly raise the standard of medical practice in India. One of the most celebrated medical practitioners of India, Sir Timelji Nariman, has said: "If Indians wish to bring into existence a profession of native doctors they should not hanker after one or two minor professorial posts in the Grant Medical College of Bombay, but should unite and set to work to found a college of their own."

CHAPTER II

DEFICIENCIES IN MEDICAL EDUCATION

Until the last few years the professorships of the various medical colleges, with few exceptions, have been held for officers of the Indian Medical Service; and personally I am strongly of opinion that most of these posts should be reserved for European I.M.S. officers for some years to come. It is, however, only fair to the various medical colleges and college hospitals, and to the medical education of the country, that officers holding these appointments should not be surrendered to the military on the outbreak of war, or for anything short of very extraordinary conditions. Such dislocation of the medical education of the country as took place during the late war should be rigidly prevented in the future. The professors have in late years been very carefully chosen from men who have more or less special training in their subjects.

It has been stated that professors are changed from one chair to another constantly to the detriment of medical education in India, and I am afraid that this charge is not altogether without foundation, as this is unfortunately still occasionally done, though it is usually for short periods only while the permanent incumbent is on temporary leave. In former years it was not an uncommon practice. During the ten years I was lent to H.E.H. the Nizam's Government I lectured at the Hyderabad Medical School on no fewer than six subjects—histology, pathology, medical jurisprudence, hygiene, theory and practice of medicine, and clinical medicine—as a rule doing two of these subjects at the same time each session; but that was a generation ago, and great advance has taken place in medical education in India since then. I am here pleading for the rigid observance of a principle; it should at this date scarcely be necessary to deprecate the switching off of officers from one professorship to another. One holds firmly that appointments to these professorships should be made solely with the object of giving the highest standard of tuition in the medical colleges and hospitals connected with them that is possible. If this cannot be done in particular cases by the appointment of I.M.S. men, then they should be open to the best men that Government can afford to secure, whether they be specialists among the members of the independent medical profession in India or anywhere in the British Empire. They should be permanent appointments and the holders should not be liable to transfer except to similar professorships in other medical institutions in the country.

The I.M.S. contains an abundance of highly qualified men for all the professorial chairs; these appointments could be filled two or three times over by suitable men of that service. Most of the I.M.S. anatomists and physiologists have filled teaching posts on these subjects or given special study to them either before entering the service or when at home on leave. The same holds good as regards medicine, surgery, pathology, midwifery, and public hygiene. Most European I.M.S. officers put in altogether one and a half to two years during their service in special education in the United Kingdom. This time is employed at post-graduate courses, expert training for specialist appointments or particular lectureships, and preparation for higher professional examinations. All this has much to do with their eligibility for professorships and higher appointments. There are few opportunities for the ordinary medical practitioner in India to attain to such high standards for teaching purposes—medical education in India has little that lends itself to such higher training after graduation, as will be shown later on.

It has been alleged by the independent medical profession in India, and put forward by them as a grievance, that the

I.M.S. has hitherto had almost a monopoly of the professorial appointments in the medical colleges and teaching hospitals. This is not strictly accurate, as there have been one or more Indian professors in each of these institutions for some years past. Allowing the contention to hold good, I am quite convinced that the preponderance of the I.M.S. has been justified, and decidedly in the interests of medical education in India—the I.M.S. officers holding these professorships were the fittest and most suitable men in India for the posts they filled. One Indian politician has remarked that "the medical colleges are dominated by the spirit of bureaucratic officialism which naturally stands in the way of working an educational institution on liberal and independent lines." I admit the first part of this contention; it has so far been very necessary to exercise firm control over the *alumni* of these institutions; it should depend upon the rate of progress of development of medical education and the direction taken by politics as to when such control can be relaxed or placed in other hands. Regarding the second part I have no hesitation in deliberately declaring that India, unaided from the United Kingdom, is not as yet sufficiently advanced to regulate and maintain the higher standards of medical education. In 1913 Sir Pardey Lukis stated that there were 150 I.M.S. officers with specialist qualifications and only eight of those were Indians; this partly explains why European officers get a larger share of the professorial posts. It is quite incontrovertible that the best men of the British medical schools will not come out to India if the professorial chairs and the better appointments go to Indians; the mere menace that this might happen has been an important factor in stopping better-qualified Europeans entering the I.M.S. during the last few years. Sir Timelji Nariman a few years ago stated: "It is only when we have a large number of teachers with hospital experience that we shall be in the position of an independent medical profession, and by perseverance, industry, and self-sacrifice we are bound to produce young men who will adorn our profession and leave names to posterity. Founding hospitals alone will not elevate our status. We must have our own college with laboratories, where some of our best men may carry on original research work. It may take years for completion, but let us make a beginning." This is from one of the foremost medical practitioners and philanthropists in India, who has founded a women's hospital in Bombay.

As will be seen, the independent medical profession claim to be able to hold the professorships on rather slender grounds. There are probably not more than a few dozen Indians with higher qualifications, whereas there were a few years ago hundreds of officers of the I.M.S. with such qualifications. I believe that the standard of medical education in India will fall in direct ratio to the extent to which European I.M.S. officers are removed from the teaching appointments. I hold a corresponding view regarding the superior posts in civil, especially civil surgeoncies—the fewer held by European I.M.S. officers, the lower will be the standard of treatment in the civil population. Suppose that all the medical professorships in India were handed over to the present independent medical profession to-morrow; what would be the result? An immediate lowering of the standard of medical education and of the tone of Western medicine, and the decline would be progressive under the conditions that now obtain. I make this statement with all seriousness and conviction. Such a proceeding would be one of the most fatal blows that could be dealt to India, the effects of which would not be fully felt in the present generation. Some may consider that in writing in this strain I am opposed to the interests and advancement of the Indian independent profession. I should be doing that part of our profession a disservice were I to write anything to encourage Indians to absorb the professorial chairs in the medical colleges and college hospitals. I have little sympathy with a cause that may possibly benefit a few dozen Indian private practitioners at the expense of the good of the whole population for generations to come, if not for all time. There are a limited number of highly talented medical practitioners among Indians, men who would make good teachers of medicine, surgery, etc., but for every one of these there are at least half a dozen in the I.M.S., and one fails to see the hardship or injustice of excluding them from the posts in Government institutions when there are equally competent Government officers to fill them.

I look upon the professorships in the colleges and college hospitals as the most important appointments in the profession in India ; they affect the higher medical education of the whole country. Once lower the standard of the expert professor's teaching and a grave step in a downward direction is taken. Any lowering of that standard will react on the whole population directly and indirectly ; the eventual result will be a lower standard of professional skill and efficiency in the treatment of the community. That the standard of medical education and practice is rising in India was vouched for by scores of reliable and responsible witnesses before the Public Services Commission and Medical Services Committee. When I recall what medical education was in India forty years ago and what it is now, I might almost state that it has developed out of all recognition ; that is all to the good, and gives hope for the future if the brake be not applied to progress.

In general terms I consider that the medical education given in the various medical colleges and schools and the hospitals connected with them is, *pro tanto*, sound and satisfactory ; in both classes of institutions, however, the education is incomplete. In some directions I believe medical education in India to be superior to that obtainable in the U.K., especially in the subjects of general medicine and surgery, and in ophthalmology and tropical medicine. Many authorities would go beyond this ; they have expressed the opinion that the general standard of medical education in India is as good as, if not better than, it is in the U.K. With this I cannot agree; there are in that education some general and many special defects. Let us enumerate a few of these, remembering that in our British, Scottish, Welsh, and Irish universities one subject is in many instances split up into several divisions, and for each division there is a special lecturer. I will take the University of Edinburgh, with which I am familiar, as an example.

Pharmacology is not taught as a special subject in any of the medical colleges. There is a vast field for investigation in connexion with the minerals and medicinal plants of India that calls loudly for scientific workers. This chair might deal with the drugs that are employed in the Ayurvedic and Unani systems, and make investigations as to any virtues they might possess; I feel that full inquiries into these drugs will bring out much useful knowledge which we have hitherto been too much disposed to ignore. It is urgently necessary that all the drugs used in these systems be thoroughly examined, investigated, and standardized on the lines of those used in allopathic medicine; all the poisons employed in these Oriental systems should be scheduled and included in a Sale of Drugs Act. All this requires a separate department corresponding to that now existing in the home universities. In the University of Edinburgh there is one Professor of Materia Medica and one of Therapeutics, and a lecturer on Experimental Pharmacology.

In our Indian universities there is one chair only in connexion with *physiology* and its different branches; in our British and Scottish universities there is one professor for what may be called general or systematic physiology and one lecturer for experimental physiology, one for physiology of the nervous system and one for histology.

It strikes one as anomalous that there should be no chair in *bacteriology*, or rather that this subject should be an appendage of the chair of pathology in the medical colleges. It should be a special chair, with all the arrangements for original research.

In Calcutta the new laboratory connected with the School of Tropical Medicine will be a help in this respect, but I am confident that it cannot fulfil all the requirements of the pupils of the Medical College, apart from the fact that it would to some extent divert the Tropical School laboratory from its original intention of dealing with tropical disease. In the University of Edinburgh there is one Professor of Bacteriology, one of General and Systematic Pathology, one lecturer on Practical Pathology, one on Morbid Anatomy, and one on Surgical Pathology.

The training in *midwifery and diseases of women and children* cannot be compared with that in our home hospitals. It is stated that from the exceptional social conditions existing male students do not get the training required, that Indian women object to men attending them in their confinement, that in the hospitals the native midwives sympathize with their sisters in this, and that students allotted particular cases are often not sent for by the midwife. I am disposed to think that the difficulties, some of which unquestionably exist, have been exaggerated. When I was a student in Calcutta, I and my contemporaries attended our full allotment of lying-in cases, and no obstacles were placed in our way, and I was told by Major-General G. G. Giffard, C.S.I., I.M.S., who had been gynecologist to the lying-in hospital for Madras for many years, that the Madras University and other students experienced no trouble regarding their attendance on the midwifery cases allotted to them. It is necessary, however, to record what others have said on this subject. Zenana hospitals, officered by lady doctors, are increasing in number and admit for accouchement some of the cases that would otherwise go to teaching lying-in hospitals. In the U.K. of course, a candidate for a qualifying examination has to show that he attended a certain number of confinements. This is theoretically the case in India, but it is not always insisted on. " In the Punjab for the M.B. examination a candidate need only attend 53 of the 80 lectures laid down for midwifery, no practical training is insisted on, and it is possible for a student to go up and pass for the M.B. degree without having seen a confinement in his life" (Sir Pardey Lukis, *Report of Public Services Commission*, vol. xii, p. 10). This man with his registrable qualification could go up for the competitive examination for the I.M.S., in England, without a day's further training; it is scarcely necessary to remark that such a partially educated man is not properly qualified to look after sick women and children (*vide infra*).

The action taken by the General Medical Council of Great Britain recently, viz. that of threatening to withdraw the privilege of registration of graduates and licentiates trained in Indian universities because the training in midwifery in the latter is insufficient, calls for a few remarks. There were, it need hardly be stated, substantial grounds for the General Medical Council of Great Britain adopting the attitude they did; the training in midwifery in India on the whole falls short of the required standards, and it is specially defective in certain provinces. That Council postponed its final decision on the question of recognition of Indian medical diplomas; it knew the social customs and the difficulties connected with midwifery training which had to be contended with, but it naturally required definite evidence "that the colleges in India had made every possible effort to raise the standard of that training before it consented to continue recognition of Indian diplomas." The fact that the Council has postponed its decision justifies the assumption that it is prepared to take the special circumstances of India into consideration.

The subject of the present and prospective conditions of obstetric training at the various centres of medical education in India has now been inquired into by Sir Norman Walker on behalf of the General Medical Council of Great Britain, accompanied by Lieut.-Col. R. A. Needham, C.I.E., D.S.O., I.M.S., Deputy-Director-General I.M.S. The report submitted to the Secretary of State for India shows clearly that "after full discussion with the authorities concerned the Indian universities are now satisfied that the means can and will be found for overcoming such difficulties as may have existed in attaining and maintaining an adequate standard of education in midwifery for the degrees which they desire to be registrable in England." [1]

There are no specialist teachers in connexion with *mental diseases*, and, so far as I was able to ascertain, there was no clinical teaching in insanity. This is a grave defect that should be remedied. In the University of Edinburgh there is a Professor of Psychiatry, and practical instruction is given at the Asylum for the Insane.

In the whole of India there is not a single "*fever*" *hospital*, notwithstanding that roughly 20 per cent. of the medical cases admitted to general hospitals are suffering from one or other form of specific fever. I am disposed to consider that there are some fevers in India regarding which it may be said we at present know nothing. It is highly probable that if we had fever hospitals with specially selected expert staffs to investigate these fevers of unknown origin, we should make some progress in their etiology. In the University of Edinburgh there is a special lecturer for Clinical Instruction in Infectious Fevers.

There are no special hospitals for the treatment of *diseases of the ear, nose, and throat*, nor are there any special lecturers on this important department of medical education. It is not possible to acquire the knowledge necessary on these subjects from the casual experience gained in the odd cases that come to the out-patients department of college hospitals for otorrhœa, nasal polypi, etc., or from the few who gain admission for such conditions as mastoid abscess.

There are no *hospitals for skin or venereal diseases*, nor are these subjects taught by special professors or lecturers. Cutaneous and venereal maladies form a fair percentage of the cases attending out-patient departments. We may possibly have still much to learn about the skin diseases of India. It is very desirable that these omissions should be remedied, both on public grounds and as an

[1] *The Lancet*, May 27, 1922, p. 1065.

indispensable part of medical education. In the University of Edinburgh there is one lecturer on Diseases of the Skin and one on Venereal Diseases.

Until quite recently there were no lectureships in connexion with *X-rays*, although all college hospitals are now provided with installations. An X-ray institute was opened in connexion with the Madras General Hospital in March 1922, which is to form a teaching centre for the whole of the Madras Presidency. There is, however, a superlatively good X-ray institution at Dehra Dun, under the expert superintendentship of Lieut.-Col. Walters, C.I.E., C.B.E. This institution has been doing splendid work for the last twenty years, and has trained many hundreds of medical men, civil and military, from all parts of the Indian Empire; undergraduates, however, are not trained there. One such institution is not sufficient for the needs of the whole of India.

The teaching of *electro-therapeutics* appears to be entirely neglected. The Great War has shown what this important branch of therapeutics can do, and it is difficult to understand how medical tuition in India has gone on so long without including this subject. The Dehra Dun Institute gives two or three courses a year on this subject to civil and military medical officers and subordinates as part of the X-ray curriculum.

There are no *dental schools* or *hospitals* in India. This will come as a surprise to many. A short course of lectures on dentistry is given at some of the colleges, and dental cases are seen as out-patients in a few of the college hospitals. There is nothing, however, in the shape of specialist education. There are thousands of dental quacks in the bazaars in India. It is strongly urged that this grave defect be removed with all possible expedition. A dental hospital was proposed in connexion with the Medical College Hospital of Calcutta some years ago, but it did not materialize. I understood that it was to have been brought before the Bengal Legislative Assembly after the War.

In January 1921 the Government of Bombay proposed to establish a dental school and hospital in the City of Bombay, and inquiries were being made as to the best way to begin. Lecturers on dentistry were attached to the Grant Medical College, Bombay, and to a few medical schools in the Presidency. This is to be followed by the institution of a dental diploma in the College of Physicians and Surgeons of Bombay.

As there are various special dental schools and hospitals, and independent dental societies granting diplomas in dentistry in the United Kingdom, this subject does not form part of the university training; in India nothing whatever of this kind exists.

There are no special hospitals for *diseases of the nervous system.* I would not lay too much stress on this deficiency, although I feel that there should be at least one hospital for these cases in each of the Presidency towns, with an expert staff attached to it. In the University of Edinburgh there is a lecturer on the physiology of the nervous system, one on psychology, and one on neurology.

Until last year there was not a single hospital for *diseases of children* in India. An excellent hospital of this kind has recently been opened in Madras; that institution owes its inception and creation largely to Major-General G. G. Giffard, C.S.I., I.M.S., the present Surgeon-General to the Government of Madras.

In the University of Edinburgh there are four clinical lecturers on diseases of children.

Last year likewise brought into existence an excellent *school of tropical medicine* with hygienic laboratory attached in Calcutta. This institution is partly supported by Government. Readers of *The Lancet* have been made acquainted with the history and progress of the Calcutta School of Tropical Medicine, which owes its inception and development to Lieut.-Col. Sir Leonard Rogers, C.I.E., F.R.S., I.M.S. This school is of inestimable value to medical education in India, and it will, it is hoped, be made use of also for post-graduate tuition.

A similar institution, the Tata School of Tropical Medicine, was to have been opened in Bombay. There has unfortunately been a sudden and unexpected interruption in the progress of the work connected with this school. It was to have been opened on April 1, 1922, and all arrangements had been made for that purpose. It was at the last moment that the Bombay Government determined to cut out of the Budget the whole sum allotted to the school and issued orders that the scheme should not be proceeded with. In consequence Sir Dorab Tata has withdrawn his offer (one lakh of rupees a year towards the expenditure to be incurred), which was contingent on the Bombay Government founding the school.

The addition of the last two institutions mentioned during the course of the last twelve months bears out what I stated at the beginning of this section, viz. that the organization and equipment for medical education in India is in process of development.

There is a very conspicuous want of arrangements for teaching the subjects connected with *public health.* As a sanitarian I was specially interested in this when on the Medical Services Committee in 1919, and went into the details. There is nothing in the organization and teaching equipment that is in the least comparable with those that exist in the U.K. in every university; those who know the arrangements made, for instance, in London University College for study of public health subjects will recognize how elaborate these have to be nowadays. I was particularly struck with the anomaly that existed in Calcutta, where the University qualifications include a diploma in hygiene and lay down a complete and severe curriculum for it, but there was at that time (March 1919) an almost complete absence of means to comply with the course. The hygienic laboratory of the Tropical School will, it is promised, be of great assistance in this respect. I was taken over this laboratory by Sir Leonard Rogers; it is very complete, especially in its research part.

The Calcutta University Commission recommended a

chair in connexion with the *history of medicine* in the Medical College; it would be specially useful to include in it the lore of Ayurvedic and Unani medicine. "It is only in the light of modern medicine that ancient systems can be judged in their true perspective and relationships."[1] The vast field covered by the history of medicine may be grasped by a review of the recent publications on the subject issued by the Clarendon Press, Oxford.[2]

Besides the deficiencies above-mentioned I would point out that there are no professors or lecturers for the training of students in applied anatomy, physiological chemistry, practical anæsthetics, tuberculosis, neurology, and other subjects which one might enumerate. All these subjects are taught by separate expert professors or lecturers in the University of Edinburgh and other universities in the U.K. In each of the colleges there are a number of Indian civil assistant surgeons who act as demonstrators and assistant professors in various subjects and seem to take the place occupied by separate lecturers in the home medical schools and universities. I have no doubt that in course of time all the deficiencies mentioned will be made good in India; the object here is to emphasize the fact that these deficiencies actually exist.

There is a complete absence of any *post-graduate training* in India. This is a lamentable gap in the education of the independent medical profession, and indeed of all branches of the profession in India. One of the most imperative requirements in India at present is the organization of regular post-graduate courses of study in the practical parts of medicine, surgery, midwifery, ophthalmology, bacteriology, malariology, and tropical medicine, X-ray, tuberculosis, etc. I believe these courses would be popular amongst both official and non-official members of the profession in India. It is of great importance to expand the facilities for post-graduate tuition in the larger hospitals and medical colleges. I look upon successful post-graduate

[1] *Report of the Cal. Univ. Com.*, vol. v, Part II, p. 107.

[2] *Studies in the History and Methods of Science*, edited by Charles Singer.

tuition as of vital significance to the progress of Western medicine; it will be specially so when India has been drained of most of its European medical officers. There should be little difficulty in arranging for these classes; there are scores of them going on all over the U.K., and hundreds of medical men are engaged in making them successful. Why this has not been methodically undertaken in India passes one's comprehension. Fitful attempts at such classes have been made on a few occasions. That is tinkering with the matter; it should be a routine part of the medical education of all the graduates, licentiates, and medical subordinates of the country. It is suggested that at any rate for the present the first step in this direction be taken by I.M.S. officers in the various medical colleges and the leaders of the independent medical profession. On my mentioning this suggestion to two of the principals of the medical colleges they stated that their professors were too busy to undertake the additional work post-graduate tuition would entail. Personally I feel that it will demand some driving power to initiate post-graduate tuition in India, and that this should at least mainly come from those who will benefit most by it—that is, the independent medical profession.

Fellowships or studentships for special research, comparable with those of the Rockefeller, British, and other Research Fellowships, would do much to further the advance of medical science and medical education; this is one of the directions in which the wealthy classes of India might give invaluable help.

The Indian Research Fund Association, which started in 1911, is one of the finest institutions of its kind in existence; until recently almost all its officers were of the I.M.S. It has carried out much important work in connexion with malaria, dysentery, cholera, kala-azar, leprosy, hookworm disease, goitre, diabetes, vitamins, and many other subjects, and I am informed encourages the members of the independent medical profession who desire to carry out any particular line of research to use the Association's laboratories. The independent medical profession should be given every possible facility in the use of these institutions.

Medical education in India had to go through its stages of incompleteness and gradual development. I would reiterate that I am in entire disagreement with those who endeavour to prove that the average medical man trained wholly in India is in professional capacity equal to the average man trained in the United Kingdom; and if we are speaking of advanced medical education, I venture to state that the difference between the best of the young graduates of India and those of the home universities is so conspicuously great that they are scarcely comparable. I was a medical student in India, in the Calcutta Medical College, and subsequently completed my medical education in Edinburgh and Guy's Hospital; later on I lectured on various subjects as previously stated; I therefore write from personal experience and knowledge. One might put the matter shortly by stating that the wide medical education obtainable in the U.K. is not available in India. I can, however, picture medical education in India, a generation or so hence, in which every branch of medical and surgical training will not only be represented, but will be up-to-date. I hold very strongly to the view that it is imperative to bring the standard of medical training both in the colleges and the college hospitals up to the level of that in the United Kingdom; to do this requires additions to the staff and equipment of the colleges and the opening out of several specialist departments in connexion with the college hospitals. India should be able to provide the sons of the soil with a first-class medical education; they should not be obliged to come to the U.K. for such an education. When colleges entirely staffed by Indians can give this education the European M.S. will have completed its task, but more than one generation will pass away before this high standard is reached.

The general impression I entertain regarding the medical training in India is that there is too much theoretical lecturing and too little actual practical work; the Indian medical student requires to be made to use his hands and his special senses on every possible occasion. We should remember that in his up-bringing he is not taught from nursery days onwards how to make things for himself; he has not played with all sorts of mechanical and other toys, nor learnt the use of simple carpenter's tools as European children do, and in this he is handicapped. His intelligence and mental powers are of a high order; his written examination papers are often wonderful productions, if we consider that he is using a foreign language. The entire environment of a medical student in the U.K. is more salutary and invigorating, and the tone of a higher standard than in the medical colleges in India; the ideals are loftier, the sense of duty and responsibility more fostered, loyalty to the profession, independence, self-reliance, and almost insensibly the principle of service to others, are engrafted—in short, the home medical schools tend to build up character better than the medical colleges in India. This is no overdrawn picture. It is what every successful Indian who has had the whole or the greater part of his medical education in the U.K. can tell us.

It is in the general finish of the training and in the special subjects that the Indian derives the greatest help in completing his medical education in the U.K. Although the minimum curriculum laid down by the General Medical Council is a five-years' course, the most highly-trained men, such as those who take the London M.D. and F.R.C.S., D.P.H., and similar inferior qualifications, do not finish their training for a period of from six to eight years, often adding materially to their efficiency by acting as house physicians, house surgeons, medical or surgical registrars in large hospitals, and demonstrators in medical schools. It is now up to the various local governments in India to see that at least their university colleges and the hospitals connected with them are organized, staffed, and equipped in such a way that they are able to give the standard of medical education obtainable in the home medical schools. This can be done and it should be done, although initially it will be rather expensive. My point is, that it should be possible for a young Indian to get a sound and complete medical education in his own country. The question of coming to the U.K. is in the majority of cases a very serious one ; the medical students of Calcutta come mostly from the middle-class people whose income just covers their expenses or falls short of this. I have been informed that corresponding difficulties are felt in the other provinces of India.

CHAPTER III

THE INDIAN MEDICAL SERVICE AND OTHER GOVERNMENT MEDICAL SERVICES IN INDIA

a. The Indian Medical Service

The organization of this service has been already referred to briefly, but it calls for a few further remarks. It is a military service with a large war reserve in civil employ. The total strength of the cadre immediately before the war was 772. At that time 475, or 62 per cent., were in civil employ, but of these 133 did not form part of the war reserve; the remainder were distributed over seven calls and available for military employ on general mobilization. There were actually 393 reverted before the end of the war; this number was altogether insufficient to meet military requirements, and as medical men could not be obtained from the U.K., a large number of temporary commissions were given to civil assistant surgeons and Indian private practitioners—in April 1919 there were 685 of these holding temporary commissions, including 354 doing duty overseas and 331 in India. The 393 I.M.S. officers embraced 197 civil surgeons, 15 officers on plague duty, 36 superintendents of lunatic asylums, 24 of the bacteriological department, and 28 of the sanitary department. The effects of such depletion are obvious. The vacancies were filled up in civil in the best way circumstances allowed —by recalling all officers from leave, and promoting civil assistant surgeons of the provincial services to civil surgeons, by private practitioners, by giving visiting charge of neighbouring districts to civil surgeons, giving civil surgeoncies in collateral charge of officers in military employ; the central jails were handed over to I.C.S. police officers, retired military assistant surgeons, or uncovenanted medical officers who had previously been in charge of jails.

Candidates for the I.M.S., after going through a two-months' training in tropical medicine, military surgery, pathology, and hygiene at the R.A.M.C. College, Millbank, proceed to Aldershot for another two months for a military course of drill, riding, hospital administration and organization, and their duties connected with the Army. Although trained militarily at Netley I did short courses both at Millbank and Aldershot in 1913 and know what an excellent finish these courses are to young men adopting a military medical career. They are then drafted to India and do a month's practical training in military sanitation and field service medical work. I understand that these young men are in future to be sent to the School of Tropical Medicine in Calcutta as soon as they arrive in India; at least this was recommended by the Medical Services Committee. They are finally sent to one of the larger Indian station hospitals. They then pass an examination in Hindustani. For promotion to captain, towards the end of their third year of service, they have to pass in medical and military organization, drill, military law, and in their duties in peace and war. There are various *voluntary* courses which they may attend in India, such as advanced bacteriology at Kasauli, the practical study of malaria at Delhi or some other suitable place, X-ray class at Dehra Dun, serology at Calcutta. The Medical Services Committee recommended that promotion from captain onwards should be on the same system as promotion in the R.A.M.C., and that every officer between his seventh and tenth year of service should undergo a post-graduate course at the R.A.M.C. College, Millbank. At the end of their second year they are eligible to apply for civil employ and then await their turn; as far as practicable they are posted to the province for which they have a predilection. The time they have to wait for civil varies with the kind of employment they seek—purely professional work such as teaching posts, civil surgeoncies ; scientific departments, bacteriology, and research ; public health, jails, or alienist departments, etc. The scientific departments posts are made by selection and according to special attainments.

The time spent in military employ, provided it is not more than five years or so, is useful to officers going into civil work. During that time they are employed in Indian station hospitals, going through the courses of study mentioned, maturing their military training, teaching soldiers first aid and military sanitation, familiarizing themselves with the language and natives, etc. The military training is valuable in grafting prompt obedience, right sense of duty and its efficient performance, accuracy, self-reliance, broad-mindedness—in short, in building up character. Much useful information regarding the present conditions of the I.M.S. not given here will be found in the Student's Number of *The Lancet*, August 26, 1922.

The I.M.S. as constituted has so far satisfied the requirements of the Government of India, but the I.M.S. has not been satisfied with the treatment it has received at the hands of Government. The Government of India, while sensible of the high value of the Indian Medical Service, for many years showed little sympathy with the reasonable expression of discontent on the part of I.M.S. officers. As the result of tension engendered by several grievances many of the trained senior officers are retiring earlier than usual and the unpopularity of the service at home has almost stopped the recruitment of the better class of men from the British schools. When I left India a few years ago the most acute discontent reigned in the I.M.S., chiefly from continuous deprivation of leave, straitened finances, and uncertainty as regards the future. The main defects of the I.M.S. were known to all concerned some years before the Great War began ; the policy of keeping down the number of officers to starvation point, which was one of the fundamental causes of discontent because it prevented men from obtaining the leave they were entitled to, was repeatedly represented. If, twelve years ago, this question had been handled in a broad-minded, statesmanlike way instead of being toyed with, the critical situation that ultimately developed might have been averted. It was a simple problem dealt with parsimoniously when liberality was indicated. The grievances of the I.M.S. have been widely published during the last ten years, and as most of them have been already removed it will serve no purpose now to resuscitate their ghosts. It will always redound to the credit of the Indian Medical Service that its officers endured their grievances patiently, silently, and with steadfast loyalty to duty throughout the war notwithstanding that in many ways the war itself intensified their causes of complaint, so as not to add to the difficulties of the medical administration during a time of strain.

Hitherto the I.M.S. has had little to knit it together as a corporate body or integral whole; the regimental medical officer considered that his primary allegiance was due to the unit to which he was attached and he identified himself with it; the men in civil had few opportunities of cultivating *camaraderie* except in their own province; such *esprit de corps* as exists in the I.M.S. has always been fostered under the most disadvantageous circumstances. One feels that the inauguration of an Indian Medical Service School in India as recommended by the Medical Services Committee in 1919 would tend greatly to unite the bonds of comradeship and common interests, and serve the important purpose of cementing the British and Indian elements of the service. In this connexion we have only to recall what Netley did for the R.A.M.C. originally and what Millbank College continues to do to-day. "The I.M.S. is a congregation of individuals held together by the common tie of similar duties, but possessing no proper central administrative department to correlate and combine the various paths of work or to which members of the service can look for advice, direction, and support."[1] There is a Director-General who represents the service with the Government, and whose recommendations until recently only reached the Council indirectly. He was not a member of the Council; his work was largely technical, yet was subjected to lay criticism. These anomalies have now been removed. It is only lately also that the embargo has been removed from his being able to see the Viceroy personally on departmental matters. The I.M.S. has greatly appreciated these concessions made in the official relations of the Director-General. The same privilege has been extended to all Inspectors-General of civil hospitals as regards their intercourse with governors of provinces and presidencies.

One of the main recommendations of the Medical Services Committee of 1919 was the conversion of the Indian Medical Service into an Indian Medical Corps officered by the present I.M.S. and transfers from the R.A.M.C., and having incorporated into it all members of the present Indian Medical Department (military assistant and sub-assistant surgeons), the Indian Hospital Corps forming its rank and file. In this scheme all British and Indian troops would be under one medical organization and controlled by one service; there would be economy in buildings, equipment, and of labour in working, wider scope for professional work, greater variety of interests for officers, and other advantages. All the arguments for and against this change were exhaustively considered before arriving at the conclusion that it was *the* solution of most of the difficulties associated with the existing organization. No other solution can be compared with this one in its completeness. Improvements of the existing organization and removal of the main grievances of the I.M.S. may tide India over the difficulties connected with one of its most intricate and complicated administrative problems, but these changes will not strike at the root of the matter, and the question will sooner or

[1] Sir George Makins, *Memorandum to the Medical Services Committee*, 1919.

later crop up again. The formation of the single organization referred to would do away with the function which has been traditional for generations. These remarks have reference to the situation that existed anterior to the inauguration of the Reforms Scheme; they have no reference to the farther complications which that Scheme introduced.

Now that the pay and prospects of the I.M.S. have been improved it is probable that when the political situation clears a certain number of Europeans who desire an Indian career will join that service if they are not required to bind themselves down to a permanent engagement under conditions that are associated with much uncertainty as to the future. There are still open to the best men from the United Kingdom many attractive posts on the civil side, especially for men with a special talent for bacteriology and research, teaching and public health work; they will find congenial work in these branches with facilities of acquiring high reputations although not affluence.

The professional standard of the I.M.S. in bygone years was probably higher than that of any existing public medical service; it is of the highest importance to India that that standard should be kept up. Thirty years ago the I.M.S. recruited the best young men turned out of our home medical schools. At that time the greater part of the high-class practice in India was in the hands of the I.M.S; in civil employ there was a substantial addition to income from this source and some men made small fortunes. Gradually since then most of the practice has been absorbed by the independent medical practitioner, thousands of whom have been trained in Government medical colleges by I.M.S. officers. The price of living has gone up progressively for many years, but especially since 1914; officers' expenses are now considerably greater than they were, and, as is well known, people live at a higher standard; these factors, of course, apply to every branch of the service.

There is at present a pronounced prejudice against

entering the I.M.S. entertained by the qualified young men of the medical schools of the United Kingdom and Ireland; they are being advised to enter the R.A.M.C., R.N., Colonial Medical Service, or accept the appointments now available at home. The main reason for its unpopularity at present appears to be the uncertainty as regards the future. It has been rumoured that "the I.M.S. is in the melting pot," or "about to be broken up," that a large number of their civil appointments will be handed over to Indian private practitioners, that the whole of their military work will be handed over to the R.A.M.C., and other legends; and a great deal of capital has been made out of the statement that as a larger number of Indians will come into the I.M.S. in the future, and that in the ordinary course of events European medical officers will have to serve under them, and there is much probability that these statements have had a deterring effect on some men who would otherwise like to come into the I.M.S. Whatever truth there may or may not be in these statements, there is one change taking place that is having a very material influence on recruitment from home, that of giving some of the professorial chairs, better civil surgeoncies, and higher civil appointments previously held by I.M.S. officers, to civil assistant surgeons and private practitioners.

Forty years or so ago Indians openly professed their earnest desire to advance by the light of Western methods. There are now crowds of Indian politicians, journalists, and medical men who claim that India no longer has any necessity to search beyond her own limits for enlightenment in the path of progress. I have already shown that as regards the profession of medicine Indians have little justification for these pretensions; in a later section it will be demonstrated that if progress is to be maintained India cannot do without the services of the best European doctors, medical research workers, teachers for her colleges, experts in public health and other branches of the medical profession.

In a speech in the House of Commons in June 1922

Lord Winterton, Under-Secretary of State for India, said "he feared he could not hold out any great hope of the possibility of greatly increasing the number of British doctors in India, but it might be possible by improved arrangements to make doctors more available, especially in scattered districts." The Medical Services Committee of 1919, foreseeing what was likely to happen under the Reforms Scheme, not only made this proposal but entered into some detail as to how it could be carried out.[1] This is a matter of serious importance for the European civil population of India.

The Government is bound within certain limits to afford gratuitous medical attendance to all their European employés, including British officers with the Army, civilians and their families, by medical men of their own race. Neglect to do this may cause such dissatisfaction as will materially affect recruitment of Europeans for all the services; in this sense therefore the I.M.S. may be looked upon as a pivotal service. "It is scarcely possible to reconcile Indian aspirations for increased employment in the medical service with the preference of European officers for treatment by doctors of their own race. It is probable that the question would become less acute with the progressive Indianization of the services under the Reforms Scheme, for it is anticipated that the officials in the larger stations will become chiefly Indian, and if Indian medical officers were appointed to these stations the difficulty would not be felt."[2]

Endeavours should be made to strike the happy mean of maintaining a sufficient number of European medical officers for our military and civil services in both peace and war, and yet dealing in an absolutely just and sympathetic way with the legitimate aspirations of Indians to hold their due place in the medical organization of the country.

1 *Report of the Medical Services Committee*, 1919, p. 34, para. 50.

2 Colonel C. Mactaggart, C.S.I., C.I.E., I.M.S., *Memorandum to the Medical Services Committee*, 1919.

I have known some Indians of the I.M.S. whose professional attainments, social habits, and other attributes removed any disqualification against their attending Europeans and their families. As a senior in military employ I have many times been obliged to settle questions where European officers' families have protested against being treated by their regimental medical officers who were Indians. It was mostly, however, in the case of young Indians whose absence of social *savoir faire* did but scant justice to their professional capacity. The whole question regarding the medical treatment of Europeans by Indians of the I.M.S. is rather complicated and to a certain extent controversial. It is dealt with *in extenso* in the Medical Services Committee's Report; it will serve little purpose to deal any further with it here.

Evidence of the growing unpopularity of the I.M.S. was years ago presented in the deterioration of the standard of candidates who appeared for the competitive examination, and the fewness of the European candidates that competed for vacancies, so that for some years past competitive examinations have ceased. When I joined the service in 1886 there were 61 candidates for sixteen vacancies. This was exceptional; the usual average then for each vacancy was three candidates. In 1913 the examiners remarked that "the percentage of failures was far greater than normal, but the answers given showed that the best men from the (home) schools were no longer competing." There was, before the war, as there is at present, a feeling of uncertainty and insecurity in the future; an air of unrest and doubt prevailed, and an apprehension that further changes detrimental to the interests of Europeans were imminent.

In April 1919 it was stated[1] that "medical students and medical men in the United Kingdom have been greatly reduced in numbers. We do not know how soon this shortage will be remedied. Medical education in

[1] *Report of the Medical Services Committee*, 1919, p. 21.

England has become more expensive, and medical aspirants and their fathers have become poorer. The Government of India will have to face keen competition at a time when in India the political balance has considerably shifted and may shift further. An Indian career occupies a position in popular estimation in England decidedly inferior to the position which it occupied in 1902. But while British competition has so much declined, Indian candidature for all Government services has greatly increased and will go on increasing." More statements of this kind are still being published, as will be seen from the following extract:

"Under existing circumstances any British candidate appointed to the I.M.S. must go out to India with prospects greatly depreciated, not only as the result of the Reforms and of the highly increased cost of living, but chiefly on account of the hostility to the British element in the service revealed in the course of the debates in the Imperial Legislative Assembly."[1] The same spirit of antipathy is, of course, manifested towards all the European services in India, the recruitment for which will thereby be greatly prejudiced.

The openings for young men at home at present are numerous and well paid—panel practice has expanded, the posts under the Ministry of Health are very attractive, health work is widening and including more men, the R.N. and R.A.M.C. are services offering men attractive and honourable careers, and there are openings in other directions. When I was a young man in impecunious circumstances I welcomed a *locum tenens* job at two guineas a week; in temporary work of this kind men now get from four to seven guineas a week.

Indians have been clamouring for a simultaneous competitive examination for the I.M.S. in England and in India. Many senior men consider this would be a serious retrograde step, and doubt whether the Indian himself fully recognizes this. It is felt that such a pro-

[1] *The Pioneer Mail*, October 7, 1921.

cedure is likely to lower the efficiency and prestige of the service. One is familiar with the various points that are advanced by Indians in favour of their demand, and with one of these many of us have much sympathy, viz. the difficulties many Indians have to surmount in going to England, especially financial, and in connexion with this the Medical Services Committee recommended scholarships. I have no doubt that it is best for himself and best for his country that the Indian competitor for the I.M.S. should go to England, anyhow for many years to come. It is not essential that graduates should take out another qualification, but it is necessary for them to complete their medical education in the U.K., and one would advise them, while they were doing so, to go through one or more of the higher examinations in medicine and surgery, or take up special subjects such as public hygiene, ophthalmology, etc. Those sent home with scholarships would have to compete (when competition is reopened) for the I.M.S.; if they failed and returned to India that country would be benefited by their higher training, which would therefore be an asset.

The attainment of the necessary standard of professional efficiency demands that candidates should have further study and hospital practice at home. Apart from the strictly professional side there are gained in the associations during this additional education a completely different professional sentiment and code of professional etiquette; more developed ideals, and higher and more venerable traditions supported by the restrictions of the Medical Act of 1858 which have not been fully developed in India so far.

Few things were more obvious to the Medical Services Committee than that the hope of obtaining civil employment was the determining factor that induced men to enter the I.M.S., and that anything which interfered with their securing work on the civil side militated against recruitment for the service. It is beyond controversy that this is the magnet that attracted the best men of the home medical schools to the I.M.S.; it is an outstanding fact, and it is folly to shut our eyes to it. An entirely military career which excludes the various opportunities afforded in civil will not attract the best-educated European medical men, although the same condition will undoubtedly appeal to young Indian medical graduates. Young European medical men desiring a purely military career would undoubtedly compete for that splendid service, the R.A.M.C. One has reluctantly come to the conclusion that the work of medical officers with Indian troops alone—that is, an uninterrupted military medical career—will never attract the highest class of Europeans, even when Indian station hospitals are ideal in construction and equipment. India requires this high class now more than ever, if the fine edifice of Western medical science which has been created by over a century of effort is not to topple to the ground. The elimination of these best men would greatly affect education in the medical colleges and schools for the worse, and I apprehend that the people would gradually, but more and more extensively, return to the faith of their fathers in indigenous systems of medicine.

On the other hand, the military side of the Indian Medical Service adds to the attraction of that service. All evidence on this point gathered from numerous competent witnesses before recent commissions and committees was to the effect that a purely civil medical service would not draw the high standard of men from the home schools who joined the I.M.S. in the early years of the present century. If we are ever again to attract good men to the I.M.S. from the medical schools of the U.K., it is beyond all dispute that they must have open to them "a mixed career—military, civil, professional, sanitary, and research, and that it shall offer varied opportunities which appeal to men of action as well as to men skilled in the different branches of the medical profession."[1]

The introduction of Indian station hospitals has altered

[1] *Report of the Medical Services Committee*, 1919, p. 27.

the essentially military part of the work of the I.M.S. for the better. From practically every point of view—organization, administration, efficiency, and convenience—Indian station hospitals are a vast improvement on the old regimental system. They have led to a higher standard of departmental and professional training in all ranks of the military medical service of the Indian Army, a progressively increasing responsibility and a wider range of executive and administrative experience in officers of the I.M.S. in military employ. Corresponding educational advantages have been conferred on military sub-assistant surgeons, who form a large part of the Indian Medical Department.

It should scarcely be necessary to emphasize the advantages from the military point of view of giving to its medical officers the benefits of civil employ and simultaneously in peace time maintaining a valuable reserve at the expense of the civil administration; and unless the Provincial Governments can show that their interests are directly sacrificed they should not object to this system. Regarding the war reserve of the I.M.S. in civil employ, Major-General Sir William Rice Edwards, K.C.I.E., C.B., C.M.G., stated in an address to the Imperial Legislative Council on March 8, 1919: "The existence of this war reserve was vital. It was the existence of this reserve that enabled the Indian divisions which proceeded overseas to go fully mobilized at the most critical period of the Empire's history." The Great War placed a very exceptional strain on the resources of the civil administration; it was excessively depleted and the standard of medical and sanitary work underwent some deterioration, but there is universal acknowledgment that no actual breakdown occurred. There were inconveniences, makeshifts and a lowering of the high standard of efficiency, but these, I submit, are among the penalties of the world's struggle experienced in every one of the belligerent countries, and they would recur in any war on the same scale. I cannot refrain from echoing the admiration felt by all who knew what the civil administration went through during the war ; the Imperial and Provincial Governments and the Indian Civil Service bore without complaint and with splendid fortitude and patience the depletion of their Indian Medical Service officers and of their best civil assistant surgeons drafted to the war.

The Public Services Commission made the following remarks on the civil and military medical organization: "From the inquiries which we made we are satisfied that under the existing arrangements, the civil medical work of the country has hitherto been economically and satisfactorily performed and that no case has been made out, either on the ground of expense or of efficiency, for ceasing to employ the war reserve of the Army in India on civil duty. If, however, it should hereafter be discovered that the medical cadre of the Army in India is insufficient to meet the civil medical needs of the administration, we consider that the Government should obtain such additional assistance as may be necessary by some form of civil recruitment to the civil medical service. Meanwhile we are satisfied that the machinery of the present system has stood the test of previous wars." Another very important conclusion arrived at was that "steps should be taken to secure that even under the gravest war conditions, the civil cadres shall not be unduly depleted, and in particular that no dislocation of the educational and scientific work of the country shall take place."

It has been contended that in other civilized countries under a constitutional government the civil and military medical services are quite separate from one another. The conditions of the medical profession are much more complicated in India than they are in other civilized countries. There are few grounds for comparison with other countries which have a homogeneous population, in which the civil medical services can readily be adjusted to meet war requirements, and in which there is only one system of medicine practised. In India there are many races, and several systems of medicine.

An opinion has been gaining ground that Indians, because they are Indians, are now being appointed to posts that have hitherto always been held by I.M.S. officers, apart from any consideration of professional merit and general suitability. I, personally, do not credit this for a moment. I am quite certain that the Imperial and Provincial Governments are dealing with an exceedingly difficult problem with equity and scrupulous attention to the present situation, and with every possible consideration for all who are concerned; I am confident that in their selection of Indians for civil posts they are choosing the very best men at their disposal.

It has been repeatedly stated by the Indian press and by Indian witnesses before commissions and committees that the higher posts both in civil and military have been denied to Indians of the I.M.S. because European officers object to serve under them. I am convinced that this does not hold good as regards the great majority of Europeans in the I.M.S. at the present day. If there have been fewer Indians in the higher appointments it is for other reasons. I have during my service several times served under Indians. If there is any foundation for such a statement it speaks ill for our training, and personally I am disposed to consider it rather libellous on our service discipline. The experience of the last few years has shown that selected Indians can hold the higher appointments, such as I.-G,, G.C.H., A.D.M.S., etc., with credit to themselves and benefit to the Government. A European who feels that he could not serve under an Indian for one reason or another must be differently constituted from the majority of us. It is morally certain that Europeans joining the service now will, in the ordinary course of things, be obliged to serve under Indians sooner or later; indeed, within the ensuing ten years, with the progressive Indianization of the services formerly almost entirely monopolized by Europeans, race distinctions will gradually die out.

I am quite certain there is no foundation whatever for the allegation that Indians do not prefer civil to military service because in civil they are given the smaller and less lucrative stations. They are treated with the most scrupulous fairness and entirely on their general merits. Administrative medical officers have been specially cautious about this. Many Indians have obtained professorships and some have reached administrative rank. That they do not do as well as Europeans is because they are not so efficient as a class—this I am convinced of after thirty-five years' work with them. If anyone has any doubt about it let him go over the professional qualifications of the Europeans and Indians in the service. I have had the opportunity of doing this officially, and I naturally have had a great deal to do with both classes of officers in my time.

The political aspirations and ambitions of India have in recent years been aroused by various factors, among which one might specially mention the publication of the Report of the Public Services Commission, the part taken by India in the Great War, and by the prodigious fillip to these ambitions given by the Reforms Scheme. The late Secretary of State for India during his tenure of office did more to foster the interests and prospects of the I.M.S. than any of his predecessors; he did all that was possible to remove the grievances under which the I.M.S. suffered. I doubt if he foresaw that the changes that are now taking place in the I.M.S. as the result of the Reforms Scheme were to prove so disastrous. As far as my service is concerned I believe it was unwise to have fixed anything in the shape of a percentage of Indians in its composition, and that it would have been better to have given Indians greater facilities for coming to the U.K. to complete their medical education and then allowing them a fair field in open competition under equal conditions with Europeans. One of the paragraphs of the Montagu-Chelmsford Report expressed the view that there should be in all services now recruited from England a fixed annual rising percentage of recruitment in India. The Medical Services Committee were unanimously of opinion that it is not advisable to attempt to fix a percentage of Indians to be admitted to the I.M.S. At the beginning of the war out of 772 officers of the I.M.S. 54, or 7 per cent., were Indians, but the number of Indians competing in the entrance examination in London had risen from 5 in 1910 to 8 in 1913 and 14 in 1914.

It would be folly to leave out of consideration the fact that the development of India on the lines of the Montagu-Chelmsford Reforms Scheme will probably call for a larger employment of Indians in the superior appointments hitherto held by I.M.S. officers, and that this will include a much larger staff of Indians for duty with the Indian Army, indeed this has been happening during the last year or so. In this connexion I am strongly of opinion that it would be decidedly premature to reduce the number of European men of the class that joined the service ten years ago. For the next generation or so India requires the best men the medical schools of the United Kingdom can supply, to develop by their influence and example the independent medical profession in India which is still in its youth.

We cannot ignore the excellent work done by a fair proportion of young T.C. Indian doctors at the front during the war; the authorities have very rightly given many of these deserving men permanent commissions in the I.M.S., and I feel sure that no European I.M.S. officer grudges this concession if those obtaining permanent commissions are sent home at Government expense to obtain the supplementary medical education that is indispensable. Much that is unfair has been stated about the inefficiency of these young Indians. It was not their fault that when they joined up they were undisciplined and inexperienced in military life. Many of them did splendid work for me during the extensive cholera epidemic in the Afghan War of 1919 and on other occasions. Our medical organization in India would have been in a much worse state than it was if they had not been available during the Great War. It is unreasonable to take a young Indian doctor, who has possibly never associated with Europeans, into the full tide of a military career without any kind of previous preparation, and expect the standard of efficiency met with in a fully trained European military medical officer. During the late stage of the Great War, as D.D.M.S., Northern Command in India, I had a great deal to do with organizing a special military medical school of instruction for these young Indians, and the results fully justified the enterprise; many of the cadets from the school became efficient medical officers and some of them were granted permanent commissions in the I.M.S.

CHAPTER IV

THE INDIAN MEDICAL SERVICE AND OTHER GOVERNMENT MEDICAL SERVICES IN INDIA (*continued*)

b. INDIAN MEDICAL DEPARTMENT

THE Indian Medical Department consists of:

1. Military Assistant Surgeon Branch;
2. Military Sub-Assistant Surgeon Branch.

1. Military assistant surgeons are recruited by competition from among Anglo-Indians and Europeans from 16 to 20 years of age. The examination, held once a year, is a trifle below matriculation standard. Candidates are chosen from those who have obtained over 40 per cent. of marks. The fewness of candidates in late years necessitated reducing the standard to 30 per cent. In Calcutta and Bombay they are provided with free quarters in the precincts of the medical colleges; in Madras they make their own arrangements, getting an allowance for quarters. They are educated at Government expense and receive a small monthly stipend. For purposes of discipline they are under a superintendent who is a senior I.M.D. officer. They are trained in drill and physical exercises by a British sergeant. On completing their final examination they are gazetted as fourth-class warrant officers. The duration of their medical curriculum is four years.

In 1914, on account of the shortage of candidates, it was determined to improve their pay and prospects, and also to change entrance competition to selection from suitable lads educated up to the test prescribed by the General Medical Council of Great Britain, thus enabling them to register as medical students; the course was also to be prolonged to five years. These changes, it was believed, would render them eligible on completing their curriculum and passing the prescribed examinations for a medical qualification registrable in the U.K. There has been a hitch in this matter of eligibility for registration.

The introduction of the Medical Degrees Act of 1916 in India made it compulsory that all military assistant surgeons should at least obtain qualifications registrable in India, and to comply with this up to the time I left India students entered for the licentiate examination of the State Medical Faculty, Bengal, the College of Physicians and Surgeons, Bombay, and the Board of Examiners, Madras. These examinations may be passed after a four-years' curriculum. This was intended to be a temporary arrangement only, and it was hoped by the beginning of 1920 to introduce the admission by nomination and a five-years' curriculum.

Military assistant surgeons are educated essentially for service with British troops and duty in British station hospitals in India, and serve under R.A.M.C. officers. The authorized strength is 739; of these, 303 are usually in civil employ and form a war reserve.

In November 1913 the strength and distribution of military assistant surgeons were as follows:

Military appointments	353
Reserve, 20 per cent.	71
Total	424
Civil appointments:	
(a) Miscellaneous	61
(b) Railways	25
(c) Ordinary civil	165
Reserve, 15 per cent.	38
Total	289

making a grand total of 713. This strength, I understand, continues.

At the beginning of the war there were 289, or 41 per

cent., in civil employment, a few only of these holding superior appointments. During the war 113 were reverted to military from civil.

The duties of military assistant surgeons in a British station hospital include those of clerk, compounder, steward, ward master, and storekeeper. They maintain discipline in the hospital and see that the orders in connexion with the treatment of patients given by R.A.M.C. officers under whom they are serving are duly carried out. They have to be on duty constantly and reside in the hospital compound in quarters provided by Government. They often hold medical charge of parties of British troops moving by road or rail from one station to another. They have small scope for actual independent professional work in station hospitals. A certain number are selected for civil employment; they then remain on probation for five years, during any part of which period the Provincial Government they are attached to may have them reverted to military duty if found unsuitable.

It is necessary that Government should have some guarantee that they are to receive some *quid pro quo* for the free training given to this class, and this is secured by insisting on seven years' service before taking their discharge, or by refunding a certain amount of the money spent on their medical education. This should not keep deserving young men of this class back if they desire to compete for the I.M.S.; in specially selected cases they should be sent home to complete their medical education and compete for that service.

All those in the military assistant branch apply for civil employment. In their selection their records of service are carefully scrutinized by the D.-G.I.M.S.; those considered eligible are put on a list and drafted into civil as vacancies occur. They first hold minor appointments for ten to fifteen years and then a certain percentage of them get civil surgeoncies. At the present time there are about forty of these officers with registrable qualifications obtained in the United Kingdom.

From personal inquiry, when on the Medical Service Committee, I ascertained that the best men are not recruited for the military assistant class because the terms of their service were not made attractive enough; those who would make suitable candidates are drafted into other branches of the Government service in which the conditions are better.

Military assistant surgeons did most excellent work in the field during the Great War. I had wide opportunities of witnessing their devotion to duty throughout that period; as compared with other services a high percentage of them were decorated or promoted for bravery or exceptionally good service.

2. Military sub-assistant surgeons are recruited by selection by the principals of the medical schools at Agra, Lahore, Madras, and Bombay (Poona and Ahmedabad), from among Indian candidates of all classes between the ages of 16 and 20, who have passed a university matriculation examination or equivalent educational test. They are enrolled, placed under military law, and the principal is their commanding officer. They are educated for service with Indian troops and normally do duty in Indian station hospitals under I.M.S. officers. The authorized strength is 894; of this number 154, who form a war reserve, may be employed in civil appointments, including miscellaneous medical charges, and semi-military posts; these appointments are much sought after and highly prized.

Military sub-assistant surgeons are educated entirely at Government expense, in the medical schools they get free quarters and a small monthly stipend. They get four years' medical training, and now, like civil sub-assistant surgeons, must enter for the licentiate examination of the College of Physicians and Surgeons, Bombay, Board of Examinations, Madras, and corresponding examinations in the Punjab and the United Provinces. On admission into the India Medical Department they are gazetted as third-class military sub-assistant surgeons and rank as warrant officers. They sign on for seven years. In an

Indian station hospital their duties are very much like those of a military assistant surgeon in a British station hospital. They are often sent in medical charge of small detachments of Indian troops moving from one station to another. They are provided with free quarters in the hospital compound. These men are loyal and valuable servants of Government whose services during the war received high commendation on all sides; a large number of them were decorated for personal bravery or promoted for excellent work and devotion to duty. Many years of my life were spent working side by side with these officers, and I left India with many pleasant reminiscences of my relations with them.

c. Civil Medical Services

The medical service of each province and local administration is under the control of the Inspector-General of Civil Hospitals or the administrative medical officer, who has under him officers of the I.M.S., civil and military assistant surgeons and sub-assistant surgeons. The number of I.M.S. officers on the permanent staffs of provinces varies from 11 in Assam to 51 in Bombay and the same number in Madras.

The Inspector-General is the head of the medical department in each province; he is responsible for the supervision of all hospitals, dispensaries, lunatic asylums and other similar institutions; and also for the supervision of medical colleges and schools. He has control of the entire medical staff and arranges for the recruitment, transfer, and promotion of the purely provincial medical personnel. He is the adviser of his Government in all matters connected with the medical administration of the province.

d. Indian Medical Service Officers in Civil Employ

The I.M.S. officers in civil employ fill the following appointments: Surgeons-General—with the Imperial Government (who is the Director-General of the Indian Medical

Service); with the Governments of Bengal, Bombay, and Madras, Inspectors-General of civil hospitals of provinces, administrative medical officers in local administrations; Public Health Commissioner with the Government of India, and a Director of Public Health with each of the provinces who has assistant directors of public health under him; civil surgeons under different local governments, professors in the university medical colleges and college hospitals, and superintendents in the medical schools, superintendents of central jails and lunatic asylums, posts in the bacteriological and research department, chemical examinerships, and a few other appointments.

e. Civil Surgeons

Civil surgeoncies are filled by officers of the I.M.S., Indian graduates and licentiates from the various universities who have been selected to be civil assistant surgeons, and military assistant surgeons selected for civil employ. European I.M.S. officers have the greater number of the civil surgeoncies, but Indians of the I.M.S., civil assistant surgeons, and Indian private practitioners with British qualifications are obtaining these appointments in larger numbers every year. The minor civil surgeoncies are held by civil and military assistant surgeons.

The work of a civil surgeon offers opportunities for specializing in various directions. These facilities have given rise to the wonderful work of Colonel H. Smith as an ophthalmic surgeon and of the late Colonel Sir Peter Johnston Freyer in litholapaxy and prostatectomy; we owe to them the classic on Indian medical jurisprudence by Norman Chevers; and one could mention many other I.M.S. officers who were civil surgeons and who have done much to advance medicine, surgery, and medical science generally. Indeed, for a man who takes an interest in his profession, the life of a civil surgeon gives him a full day's congenial work every day. It is not now as lucrative as it was in bygone years, but it is work that can give much satisfaction, contentment, and happiness, and these are greater blessings to a man than affluence. With the enhanced rates of pay recently granted even a family man should now be able to live fairly comfortably and free from financial cares. A small proportion of civil surgeons, especially those of presidency towns and capitals of provinces, do still make considerable additions to their incomes in fees.

The duties of the civil surgeon have been widening year by year and are now to a large extent supervisional and administrative; his chief work, however, is, as it should be, in the hospital. He is doing a much larger amount of work for Government than formerly; there is decidedly less time for private practice and consequently his income from this source has greatly lessened.

The relations between the various branches of the civil medical department have been, and continue to be, harmonious. Some of my most agreeable experiences when accompanying civil administrative medical officers on their rounds have been in seeing the real sympathy they have with their Indian assistant surgeons, which was fully reciprocated. This is some proof of the fibre of these senior I.M.S. officers who manage to keep these men of diverse temperament, training, associations, and views together as members of one large family; they, by the lessons of experience, know that there must be mutual concessions to keep the machinery running smoothly.

f. Civil Assistant Surgeons

The civil assistant surgeon branch is open to all classes of Indians, Europeans, and Anglo-Indians; there have been but few candidates among the latter two classes in late years.

Candidates for appointment are selected according to their position at their final professional examination at the university, or by a separate competitive examination, or by nomination to fill vacancies or fresh posts on the temporary establishment. They are all passed students of one or other medical college, and are either graduates (M.B.) or diplomates (L.M.S) of one of the universities. On permanent appointment they execute a bond to serve the civil Government for five years, or in default pay a fine of Rs. 500. They are not bound to serve with troops. The total number of civil assistant surgeons is 685; the number in the provinces varies from 49 in Assam to 232 in Madras. A certain number of the first-class civil surgeoncies are reserved for them, and many hold minor civil surgeoncies. Some are employed as lecturers at the medical schools, demonstrators and assistant professors in the colleges, as house surgeons and house physicians in the college hospitals and other large hospitals, in charge of hospitals at headquarter stations and the larger rural dispensaries. In addition various railway appointments, posts as medical inspectors of schools, assistants to chemical examiners, and a few other appointments are held by them.

The evidence brought before the Medical Services Committee indicated that the class of civil assistant surgeon "lays claim not only to the superior appointments now open to military assistant surgeons but to a large proportion of those held in each province by members of the I.M.S." They assert that their class is, as shown in the recent war, perfectly able to take the place of the I.M.S. officer and of the military assistant surgeon as a war reserve. No impartial judge familiar with the facts could accept these contentions; into this subject it is undesirable to enter here. The Public Services Commission and Medical Services Committee made several important suggestions for improving the conditions of this service, almost all of which have, I believe, been given effect to.

g. Civil Sub-assistant Surgeons

The civil sub-assistant surgeon branch is open to all classes of Indians who are matriculates of a university or hold a corresponding certificate of general education. They are educated in the provincial medical schools, the superintendent of which is principal and selects the candidates for entrance. The medical course is four years. A considerable number of them receive Government scholarships or scholarships from local fund sources during their training, but many defray their own expenses. Government does not bind itself to accept its scholars, but selects the best. They are recruited to fill vacancies or fresh appointments on the temporary lists. Selected sub-assistant surgeons are eligible for promotion to assistant surgeon after twenty years' service. When permanently engaged they sign on for service under the Provincial Government for five years, and undertake if necessity arises to serve in military duty in any part of India. A heavy fine is imposed for breach of this bond.

There are 3,442 civil sub-assistant surgeons holding permanent appointments in India, besides which a considerable number are on a temporary list in each province. They form a highly important part of the medical service in the provinces, and carry out the bulk of the work in treating the poorer classes of the country. They are as a class sound in professional knowledge, faithful in the discharge of their duties, and greatly appreciated by the people. They are just the type of medical men required in the rural areas. Five or six times the existing number could be employed with immense advantage to the medical work of the country ; but this is another question, and I here merely throw out the hint to our administrators in India ; those who are thoroughly familiar with our requirements as regards medical personnel will bear out my statement.

Civil sub-assistant surgeons in charge of small hospitals and dispensaries in the districts are rather isolated from communication with their professional brethren. They do most useful work. There is little to stimulate their professional ardour. It would be advantageous to the medical service to which they are attached and to themselves to ensure their being transferred to larger towns and hospitals periodically and to grant them periods of study duty to enable them to go through refresher courses of professional work.

Their duties vary. They are placed in sub-charge of police, jails, lunatic asylums, and state railway hospitals; they hold independent charge of local fund, canal, and itinerating dispensaries, and serve as travelling medical subordinates on State railways and with survey and forest parties, and have to deal with outbreaks of epidemic disease occurring in the vicinity of their charges. The pay and conditions of service in all provinces are more or less identical.

Civil sub-assistant surgeons are anxious to be put on the same footing as civil assistant surgeons, both as regards medical education and status. They have no reasonable grounds to support this claim. It would be a fundamental administrative mistake to change their status. India requires men of just their standard—wants many more thousands of them—and, as at present constituted, they form an indispensable part of the medical organization of the country.

CHAPTER V

THE INDEPENDENT MEDICAL PROFESSION IN INDIA

THE composition of the independent medical profession in India has been already briefly dealt with, and it will have been seen that the manner of its growth has been largely influenced by the directions in which medical education has developed. The result is the formation of a body of medical practitioners varying extremely in professional attainments. The independent medical profession here referred to, however, comprises the graduates and licentiates of the various universities, Indians who have in part or entirely completed their medical training in Europe, and the large body of men trained as civil assistant surgeons and sub-assistant surgeons (civil and military) who have left the Government service or were not selected for permanent employment in it.

At the present time the independent medical profession is overstocked in the large towns, while there is starvation as regards medical relief in the smaller towns and villages, and the outlying districts generally. As years roll on, this disparity will increase unless some radical change occurs in the distribution of medical men. Indeed, the prospects of the ordinary Indian private practitioner in the earlier years of his professional career in cities and large towns are very limited at present, and the path which leads to success is not very smooth. The experience of the last fifty years has shown that no matter how many medical men are trained and turned out of our medical colleges in India, they will not go into the districts and practise where hospitals and dispensaries have not been established by district boards or municipalities or the provincial governments.

The inhabitants of rural areas will not or cannot pay the fees demanded by graduates or licentiates of the universities, or even those asked by diplomates of the various medical schools. The serious difficulty that has arisen will be readily understood by the following table compiled for the Calcutta University Commission in March 1919 :

	Number practising in Calcutta.	Number practising in Bengal, outside Calcutta, and in Behir and Orissa.	Number engaged on special estates (tea gardens, jute mills, coalfields, etc.)	Number practising in Assam.	Total.
Holders of English Medical Degrees .	76	43	—	—	119
Holders of Indian Medical Degrees or licences qualifying for the rank of assistant surgeon . .	433	435	11	1	880
Registered practitioners of the sub-assistant surgeon class . . .	211	1,633	69	22	1,935
Total . . .	720	2,111	80	23	2,934

The population of Calcutta is roughly a million ; that of the rest of Bengal and of Bihar and Orissa is seventy-nine millions. " Leaving out the holders of English medical degrees, and the small number of other men employed on special estates, we see that there is one medical graduate or qualified practitioner of the assistant surgeon class for every 2,300 persons in Calcutta, and only one for every 181,000 persons outside Calcutta. Of the sub-assistant surgeon class there is one for every 4,700 persons in Calcutta and one for every 48,000 persons outside Calcutta. The region outside Calcutta includes Dacca and the other towns in Bengal, and Patna and other towns in Bihar and Orissa. The number of registered practitioners (of both classes) is one for 1,550 persons in Calcutta, and one for 38,000 for Bengal outside Calcutta and Bihar and Orissa." The same conditions prevail in other parts of India, although less pronounced, as rural Bengal is more densely populated than other country areas.

In November 1913 there were on the Medical Registers of Great Britain and Ireland 40,913 medical practitioners; the population of Great Britain and Ireland was then forty-five millions—roughly one doctor to every 1,100 persons. At that time the population of India was over three hundred millions; therefore there would have to be six times the number of Indian independent medical practitioners there were in Britain and Ireland to come up to the English standard; that is to say, 250,000 independent practitioners could be utilized in India. In 1913 there was no Medical Registration Act in operation in India, but so far as could be ascertained there were about 1,771 independent medical practitioners at that time holding registrable qualifications.[1] It is probable that the number of independent practitioners was much underestimated; but even allowing that there were three or four times the number stated it is obvious that India requires many thousands more doctors. Government service and Government institutions cannot be expected to deal with the whole of the medical needs of India, and one is convinced that more and more of the work of medical relief must be undertaken by unofficial bodies and private agencies. This principle has already been accepted and is being given effect to by the opening of more private hospitals.

The I.M.S. has done a great deal towards elevating the tone of the medical profession as practised by Indians during the last seventy years; but the raising of standards in a whole country is the work of many generations, and much in this direction has still to be done. To set this standard demands medical men of the highest repute and character, and if they are not forthcoming there will be progressive deterioration. The lower type of medical man who fails to get into other branches of the medical services in India is not the one either to maintain or raise the standard; it would be years before the full measure of the evil effects of admitting such men would be disclosed.

[1] Sir Pardey Lukis in *Report of the Royal Commission on the Public Services in India*, vol. xii, pp. 9 and 18.

It will then become patent to all—there will be a hideous awakening, and, if better councils then prevail, a reaction. It does not require a prophet to foresee this; it will be an obvious example of cause and effect. One earnestly hopes that action will be taken in time to ward off this catastrophe; this one pleads for in the interests of the people of India, and not in those of the I.M.S. British rule in India has effected great changes for the better in the general health conditions of the people of that country, and it has introduced the great blessings of modern medicine and thereby saved millions of lives and relieved suffering in many millions of people; those who jeopardize these priceless privileges accept a very grave responsibility, and future generations will not readily forgive them for doing so.

In developing the independent medical profession the creation of medical colleges in the presidency towns and the capitals of the provinces, with the erection of public hospitals by voluntary subscription, would go a long way. The independent profession would then have many specialist chairs and hospital appointments at their disposal. The College of Physicians and Surgeons of Bengal referred to has on its staff some of the best private Indian medical men in Calcutta.

The efforts made by the independent medical profession in India to capture a few professorships of the Government medical colleges from the I.M.S. have always appeared to me to be somewhat lacking in dignity. One is perfectly convinced that if the colleges and hospitals alluded to above were started, a generous rivalry would spring up between them and the official colleges which would be of the greatest value to both groups of institutions. This would be a broad-minded way of meeting the urgent needs of the independent profession in India; obtaining a few Government professorships in the official colleges is the narrow way that has in it no progress, and may be a means of materially interfering with medical education in the country. The sooner this broader view is accepted the better it will be for the sick poor, the medical education of the country, and for the peace of mind of the independent medical profession. This will have to be done some day if there is to be any material progress in the independent medical profession. It is actually happening on a small scale in Calcutta at the present moment. India requires thousands more medical men of higher and lower grades ; there appear to be a want of a sense of proportion, and perhaps some degree of selfishness in railing against a few hundred I.M.S. officers holding appointments on the civil side, especially as these men are the pillars keeping up the standard of medical education and of medical and surgical treatment in the country. How are the hospitals and medical colleges in the U.K. built and maintained ? Government has practically nothing to do with their creation ; occasionally, and then only when public hospitals are in straitened circumstances, Government makes an allotment ; one feels that the Governments of provinces would similarly come to the help of any properly organized and efficient public hospital in India supported by voluntary contributions. No Government in the world has been more generous in meeting the demands for more hospitals and the support of them than the Government of India. How has the School of Tropical Medicine in Calcutta just erected been provided for ? Mainly by private philanthropy.

In the United Kingdom there are thousands of people perpetually engaged in collecting subscriptions for the public hospitals and thousands of doctors give their services free to the sick admitted into these institutions. There is great wealth in India, though it is irregularly distributed ; could not some of it be diverted to the erection of more hospitals and medical colleges and schools ? Millions more people are in need of medical relief ; will the rich men of that country continue to refuse to provide it ? It is, one feels, up to the independent medical profession in India to initiate measures to tap this fertile source of latent philanthropy ; the wealthy classes, I feel confident, will do what is required of them if the independent medical profession presents their case wisely and unselfishly and with the object of developing the means of affording medical and surgical relief to the poor who cannot afford to pay for advice. The object in view can only be carried out by widely extended continuous effort, some self-sacrifice, service to others, and sympathy with the sufferings of our fellow-creatures. One would appeal to the educated classes of India to make this effort, and at the same time warn them not to be disappointed with slow progress. Those medical men who enter this arena should do so on humanitarian grounds, unselfishly, and without expectation of personal reward except the gratification of knowing that they are doing well for their country. The suggested endeavour, however, opens to the independent medical profession in India a noble theatre of future professional enterprise, and the dayspring of a new era.

In Bombay there are several large voluntary hospitals—the Parsi General Hospital, Dr. Masina's Surgical Hospital, Sir Timelji Nariman's Lying-in Hospital, and in Calcutta there are likewise a few. More institutions of this kind are required in practically all cities and larger towns of the country.

It would be well for Indian statesmen, newspaper proprietors and editors, merchants, landowners, philanthropists, doctors, lawyers, schoolmasters, ecclesiastics of all kinds, their wives and daughters, to review what is being done in the United Kingdom and in the United States year in and year out in connexion with the medical work of their nations, including medical institutions and medical education. They are perpetually and strenuously organizing large and small charities for medical relief for their countries as a whole, and for their towns; they are unceasingly engaged in Red Cross work and in labours of social science. What is needed in India is a wider human sympathy, more energy, greater thoughtfulness regarding the suffering poor, and a recognition by Indian philanthropists that hitherto they have done little to supply this, and a firm and universal resolve to make amends in the future for their omissions in the past.

Early this year Lady Reading started a new fund in the hope of promoting a wider distribution of skilled medical aid for the poorest classes of Indian women and children, part of the fund being intended for the Hardinge Medical College for Women in Delhi, which is doing such splendid work in the training of women students to be doctors. When opened this fine College was not complete; additional buildings had to be constructed, and the attached hospital completed; and the two lakhs of rupees a year granted by Government are insufficient to meet the requirements. The College, which was opened three years ago after much thought and labour to bring the blessings of Western medicine to many more thousands of suffering women and children than receive them, now calls loudly for additional support, and this help should come from all parts of India, as the students are admitted from all quarters of that country. A very serious point is that the hospital has still too few beds to secure affiliation to the Punjab University as a teaching hospital. A further object of this new fund is to establish an All-India Nursing Association for Indian women on the same lines as the Lady Minto Association for European women in India. There is in this and other fields unlimited scope for the energies of Indian ladies by the exercise of their influence to encourage their countrywomen to enter a sphere of usefulness that is specially theirs, and to collect subscriptions.

Several of the Provincial Governments of India in consequence of their crippled financial state (a result of the war) have been obliged to deplete their medical budgets and cut out many of their intended medical and sanitary works; some hospitals have been compelled to reduce the number of beds, which is always a melancholy procedure. Might one here venture to appeal to wealthy Indians to come to the help of their Provincial Governments in these matters?

The Indians of the independent medical profession appear to have wide and vague aspirations without the initiative necessary to give them practical expression. A conglomeration of races such as that of India that yearned to create a really great independent medical profession would long ago have acted more and talked and grumbled less against the Government and the I.M.S. It would have gathered large funds by voluntary subscriptions, got the best architects to plan and the best engineers to build up-to-date public hospitals, and medical colleges and schools to train their young men, sent selected men home to study and work out the best forms of medical education to impart, and got the help of the Royal Societies, universities, and medical schools in their enterprise; given liberal scholarships to dozens of men to go to the U.K. for special training as experts in the subjects they had a natural penchant for, and subsequently converted these scholars into demonstrators and professors or lecturers in the medical colleges and schools. It is not too late. If they begin now they will in the course of ten to twenty years' time reap the first-fruits of their labours.

Many private practitioners urge the development of the independent medical profession in India, and consider that this can be fostered by replacing I.M.S. officers by Indians recruited entirely in India. How the replacement of some of the I.M.S. in civil by private practitioners is going to affect the growth and development of the independent medical profession is not made quite clear by the Indians who advocate it, the proposal merely changes one set of *officials* for another.

If the present districts are split up into smaller ones more civil surgeons will be required, and it seems desirable that these additional appointments should be given to Indians, especially as the great majority of the new sub-district staffs are Indians.

Under the altered circumstances, and with the progressive increase of official work and higher efficiency demanded, it is not easy to see how Government can justify the attitude of having a fixed and unchangeable number of appointments in the I.M.S. and in the civil medical department generally. The work, because of the advance of knowledge in medical and sanitary service, has grown enormously, yet the authorized number of medical men employed on the civil side has remained much the same for the last quarter of a century.

There are many who feel, as I do, that the civil medical organization should be extended, and that, supplemented by charitable medical organizations, efforts should be made to get into touch with wider and wider areas, so that medical relief might be available to the millions in villages who now do not get it. More medical officers and a vastly larger subordinate medical staff and more hospitals are called for throughout the country. There are, however, limits to the capacity of the Government of India to place the benefits of Western medical relief at the disposal of the enormous population.

It is universally recognized that the quality of Indian medical men has greatly improved, and this applies not only to those educated in the United Kingdom, but also to those trained in India. As already stated, there is a greatly increased number of these men and it is desirable to consider how employment can be found for at least some of them. One direction in which Government can come to the rescue is the creation of a larger number of civil surgeoncies.

It is almost unanimously stated by Indian private practitioners that officers of the Indian Medical Service have been encroaching on their practice. It is difficult to understand how they arrive at this conclusion; everything points to the reverse. One of the causes lessening the attractiveness of the I.M.S. is the loss of income from private practice that has taken place because of the growth of the independent medical profession, which has now absorbed a great portion of the practice I.M.S. officers held in former years.

A great change has come over India in respect to private practice. Years ago, when I.M.S. officers had no competitors in private practice, and when their executive duties were much lighter than now, most of them enhanced their incomes to a satisfactory extent by private practice. At present it is only the more highly talented and those with special facilities who make exceptionally large incomes from fees. The idea appears to prevail in the United Kingdom that fortunes are still made by many I.M.S. officers in civil employ. That this is not the case was most forcibly shown by Sir Pardey Lukis in 1913, in his evidence before the Public Services Commission. "The actual figures as regards posts classed as practising appointments show that the competition with the private practitioner is almost negligible when the vast population is taken into consideration." The estimated average amount from fees received by Indian Medical Service officers in civil employ was Rs. 317·8 a month. Only those who have not considered the facts can allege that the I.M.S. in civil employ has checked the growth and development of the independent medical profession in India. In the year just mentioned there were only 196 I.M.S. officers in practising appointments among three hundred millions of people. The fee of the I.M.S. civil surgeon is Rs. 10 in two of the presidencies and Rs. 16 in the other, that of the average Indian private practitioner is from 4 to 8 rupees (but goes as low as 1 or 2 rupees); the fee of the European civil surgeon is too high for the vast majority of Indians; hence he is only called in occasionally in emergency or in consultation.

Were the practitioners of the independent medical profession of the same calibre as European I.M.S. officers, it would be morally impossible to prevent the submergence of the latter as regards private practice; the European medical officer would certainly lose all practice amongst Indians, and, with the exception of a small number required for the non-Indian community and the British troops in the country, would in all probability in time disappear altogether.

A progressively increasing number of Indian graduates and licentiates will multiply the private practitioners in the larger towns, and swell the number of competitors for the Government provincial services and local municipalities. This, as past experience has demonstrated, will materially decrease the income of Government officers holding superior appointments from private practice, while it must decrease that of Indian private practitioners themselves.

The I.M.S. has practically created the independent medical profession in India and has done much to foster its growth and development. In the large towns, where the advantages of Western medicine are recognized, a most useful and powerful body of private practitioners is forming. They do not appear to take in all the disadvantages associated with an official service. They have their freedom of action and opinion, an asset the high value of which they do not appear to recognize. It is only men who have been bound by the four corners of a series of red books for the greater part of a lifetime who can fully prize the vast privilege of reasonable liberty of professional opinion and action.

Private practitioners complain that they suffer from want of hospital experience after graduating. I have a certain amount of sympathy with them in this. They clamour for house physiciancies and house surgeoncies, and for posts as honorary physicians and honorary surgeons in the larger hospitals. I have no doubt but that young graduates and licentiates just about to begin practice would be greatly benefited professionally by being attached to our larger hospitals for a period.

Some experienced I.M.S. civil surgeons are not satisfied that the creation of honorary physicians and surgeons in our larger Government hospitals would be altogether successful, and I am rather doubtful as to whether private practitioners could be advantageously introduced into official teaching hospitals as members of an honorary staff; if such appointments were not a success they might possibly militate against the working of these institutions. As regards honorary physicians and surgeons in non-teaching hospitals, it is only fair to state that this system was on trial in Bombay in the military hospitals for Indian troops during the war, and after close inquiry I learnt that it was a most successful experiment; I personally saw several senior practitioners working in these institutions day after day; they brought the highest skill to the treatment of the men and did their work conscientiously, and this had gone on for years in the same satisfactory way. The conditions are somewhat different from what would be the case in our larger mofussil hospitals; those so employed were mostly Hindus and Parsis, and one felt that there was a sort of *esprit de corps* in operation; it is quite possible that there would not be the same success in peace time in the large hospitals of up-country towns.

Taking all points into consideration, I should be disposed to allow private practitioners to have all the advantages reasonably obtainable from State hospitals and other medical institutions so long as this does not interfere with the machinery of routine work.

I am strongly of opinion that all the college hospitals should appoint house physicians and house surgeons from among the most successful students each year, irrespective of whether they intend to enter Government service as assistant surgeons, compete for the I.M.S., or go into private practice. I disapprove of the custom of posting civil assistant surgeons to college hospitals to fill these appointments for one or two years. The adoption of the principle advocated in all the larger and smaller hospitals connected with medical training—including in it young graduates and licentiates and military assistant surgeons just qualified in the college hospitals, and military and civil sub-assistant surgeons in the hospitals connected with the medical schools—would raise the standard of medical and surgical work in India. These appointments should be limited to three, or at the outside six months, so that four or at least two groups of young qualified men get these posts each year; they should while so employed be provided with free quarters in the hospital and receive a subsistence allowance, but be excluded from private practice.

There are indications that local bodies, district boards and municipalities, which at present employ Government medical officers, may in the future seek to replace them by private practitioners recruited by these bodies, in which case the actual provincial cadres of medical officers run the risk of being much reduced. At the present time the dispensaries and hospitals in the districts and capital towns are under the control of district boards and municipal committees, and the medical institutions are supervised by committees.

It has been urged that there is no need for a Government medical service, that each local or district body should make its own arrangements by employing private practitioners for the treatment of its sick, engaging these practitioners for a certain number of years by contract. This would mean that all outlying and unpopular districts would get no medical relief, as there would be no candidates for them. The Public Services Commission's Report states: "We are satisfied that in the present conditions of India, if there were no State service there would be large tracts of country which would be left without any regular provision of medical relief. We are also convinced that State control is necessary in order to secure the continued and extended diffusion in India of Western medical knowledge. We have no hesitation, therefore, in finding that a State service is needed and to this extent approve of existing arrangements." With this statement I am in full agreement.

One of the most urgent administrative problems in India is that of providing adequate medical relief for the people. It has been estimated that a hundred million people of our Indian Empire live and die beyond the reach of the simplest Western medical aid. The wide area of work that this lays open speaks for itself. Yearly, as the result of the growth of Western methods, other fields are being unfolded, such as the sanitary welfare of the people, saving of life and suffering amongst women and children, reduction of the incidence of malaria, tuberculosis, etc. Every advance in scientific knowledge throws additional work and responsibility on the Government of India—the epoch-making discovery of Sir

Ronald Ross regarding the relationship of mosquitoes to malaria, the treatment of cholera by intravenous injections of hypertonic saline solution introduced by Sir Leonard Rogers, the emetine treatment of dysentery, are a few examples; the fields opened out in these alone are considerable, and if they are taken advantage of fully, will save hundreds of thousands of lives and relieve suffering in many millions. It is remote from my intention to harrow the feelings of the reader with reference to the sufferings of the people for want of adequate medical aid, but I cannot refrain from dwelling on one aspect of the subject, the infant mortality.

The most lamentable phenomenon in medical statistics in India is the appalling infant mortality, due partly to economic and social conditions, and partly to the practices adopted by *dhais* or indigenous midwives. "The description of the revolting practices of these women would appear incredible to anyone who is not acquainted with India; but, unfortunately, it is too true and the state of affairs which prevails is a reproach to the country."[1] I can bear personal testimony to this statement, and as a matter of fact have recorded numerous instances of these barbarous practices. The Sanitary Commissioner with the Government of Bombay[2] stated that the rate of infantile mortality in the City of Bombay is possibly the highest in the world, and is not confined to the poorer classes. "After every allowance has been made for various sources of fallacy," says the Commissioner, "the infantile mortality cannot be fairly estimated at less than 500 (per mille), which means that of every two infants born one dies before reaching the age of twelve months." It is inexpressibly regrettable that a more vigorous effort is not made by the Indian community itself to prevent this overwhelmingly sad tragedy. "Attempts through the agency of Victoria Memorial Scholarships and other bodies to effect an improvement in the training of *dhais*

[1] *The Pioneer Mail*, May 13, 1922.

[2] *Report of the Sanitary Commissicner to the Government of Bombay*, 1920.

have produced beneficial results. Progress is necessarily slow. The women are ignorant and jealous of their hereditary rights, and require an immense amount of tact and patience on the part of the teacher. Centuries-old customs die hard in India, and there is no great demand for a superior class of attendant."

Maternity and infant-welfare schemes are in operation in Bombay, Madras, Calcutta, Delhi and several large towns, and on the whole they are doing a certain amount of good. They are not as popular as in Western countries. The Health Officer of Calcutta has lately stated : " Poverty, bad housing conditions, overcrowding and underfeeding, child marriage and the *purdah*, play an important part in undermining the health of the mothers with the result that a large number of weakly and immature babies are born only to die. 'Dirty midwifery' is another cause of the high death-rate among newly-born infants. The maternity centres in Calcutta have done most valuable service, but unfortunately the opposition offered to health visitors by many people of the poorer classes is still a serious obstacle."[1]

The Countess of Dufferin's Fund Committee, which is doing such valuable work for India, has recently placed two lady doctors on special duty to inquire " into the conditions of women industrial workers during child-birth. It is believed that many facts will be elicited which will be of great service in reducing maternal and infant mortality in all classes of life in all parts of India."[2]

The Indian Government has done a vast amount of medical work and is expanding it yearly. It is the only civilized government in the world which provides for the medical and surgical wants of the entire population and the education of practically the whole medical profession in Western medicine. I suggest that the time has come when the people must do things for themselves, build more hospitals, create more medical colleges and medical

[1] *The Lancet,* July 14, 1922, p. 95.
[2] *British Medical Journal,* April 29, 1922, p. 695.

schools with their own funds and under their own organization; these might be State aided and guided, until they are self-supporting and are found to be working under satisfactory conditions and with assured efficiency.

Co-operation with non-official medical institutions and private medical practitioners appears to me to be one of the directions in which medical relief can be considerably extended. One special direction in which such co-operation appears to be possible is with the medical missionaries' hospitals and Salvation Army medical institutions. I feel convinced that it is possible to effect a much larger degree of co-operation than has hitherto been adopted between civil hospitals and mission hospitals, and that such co-operation would be much to the advantage of the sick who are unable to pay fees. There are about 330 medical missionaries, men and women, in India, connected with their hospitals and doing a great deal of most excellent medical and surgical work in a silent and unostentatious way. There is at present some want of sympathy shown regarding missionary medical work; this, I believe, would disappear with a better mutual understanding. In the interests of the suffering poor we require cordial co-operation and a warmer and more united sympathy. Is it not possible for Government to give assistance to these missionary hospitals, if necessary making the amount of the donation bear a proportion to the amount of medical and surgical relief given? Grants-in-aid to these and other non-official hospitals, if made with the necessary safeguards, would set in motion a very economical means of materially extending the medical relief of the country. I have for many years witnessed the wonderful medical and surgical work done in many of the Church Missionary Society's Hospitals and American Mission Hospitals. During the late war we employed many of their doctors and used their hospitals. Addressing the local municipal conference at Tinnevelly on July 26, 1922, Major-General G. G. Giffard, C.S.I., I.M.S., urged the need for a concentrated effort to co-ordinate medical activity in the Madras Presidency and recommended that a complete survey should be made of the hospitals and dispensaries in each district and their work reorganized in such a manner as to prevent overlapping. "Medical institutions," he said, " were scattered about without any definite plan, with the result that in some towns there were hospitals owned by Local Boards and missionary bodies which kept up a perpetual rivalry. In one district there were eleven dispensaries in one of which only twenty persons were treated for minor ailments. He asked the conference to help the Government by reorganizing the work of hospitals and dispensaries in such a manner as to make better use of the existing staff and get a better return for their money."[1] The sound advice given by General Giffard might with great advantage be followed in the other presidencies and provinces.

I would suggest other ways in which the co-operation of the independent medical practitioner might be sought in carrying out the medical relief of the poorer classes.

Would it not be possible to subsidize some private practitioners, in small, outlying districts, to extend the benefits of Western medicine to these areas, the subsidy being in course of time withdrawn, when a form of rural medical practitioner was established in the country? It may be remembered that this is what has been done in some of our colonies. The special object of this suggestion is to endeavour to extend medical aid to centres hitherto without it; the young Indian private practitioner could fill a huge hiatus in this direction. It is recognized that careful supervision of such work would be necessary. It will at once be objected that the rural population in India is too poor to pay the fees of medical practitioners. There are in rural districts, however, wealthy *zamindars* as well as thriving *ryots*, and, so far as I am aware, no really strenuous efforts have been made to test to what extent these could conjointly support medical practitioners in district areas. Surely such an experiment is deserving

[1] *The Pioneer Mail*, August 4, 1922.

of trial! In this way, it seems to me, many hundreds of young medical men might get employment, and many thousands of sick now untreated would obtain relief.

The development of the independent medical profession in India is to some extent kept back by the faith which a very large proportion of the people have in the ancient systems of medicine, by the overcrowding of the profession with a mass of defectively educated and trained men issuing from several unrecognized medical schools, and by the packing of the larger towns with young Indian doctors who will not attempt to practise in the smaller towns, villages, and remote districts. To these causes may be added a certain amount of abuse of State hospitals with free treatment by persons in good circumstances.

I share the sympathy which most of my contemporaries feel for the Indian private practitioner; we have seen him developing under circumstances that were not altogether favourable, and we have considerable admiration for many of his characteristics; we have had a great deal to do with his growth and progress. Nevertheless we who have given the greater part of our life in service to India cannot blind ourselves to what is obvious, that the average man of the independent medical profession in India is a long way, possibly a few generations or so, behind the standard of his British confrère in the United Kingdom. Guided on right lines he may eventually attain to that standard.

One earnestly hopes to see in the future a civil provincial medical cadre in each part of India, giving a wider field of employment to young graduates and licentiates from the Indian medical colleges, and an extension of the blessings of allopathic medicine to district areas and villages that hitherto have had no such privilege. The healing work required is well-nigh limitless, and extensions of it should be considered in connexion with utilization of the services of private practitioners and practitioners of the ancient systems who have been trained at least partly under our guidance as suggested later on.

CHAPTER VI

PUBLIC HEALTH WORK IN INDIA

THE public health services consist of those connected with the Army in India, and those of the civil administrations; they are quite separate. The sanitary organization of the Army consists of the D.M.S. in India, who advises the Commander-in-Chief on all questions affecting the health of the troops; he has on his staff an A.D.M.S. (Sanitary). Each division has its divisional sanitary officer, and each battalion has a medical officer attached to it for sanitary duties. Each combatant unit has its regimental sanitary detachment. The sanitary work of the Army in India calls for no further remarks; I consider it to be one of the best parts of our administration in that country.

The organization of the public health services in the civil administration has, during the last two or three years, been simplified and rendered more efficient. The present organization may be briefly stated to consist of a Central Board of Health at Imperial Headquarters, composed of the heads of the medical, public health, and research departments, and a Board of Health in each province. Each province has a Director of Public Health and several Assistant Directors of Public Health; health officers are employed by the larger towns, each of which has its own sanitary inspectors.

The following are the changes made recently in the organization of the Imperial and provincial sanitary departments. A Central Imperial Board of Health for India has been established, the Sanitary Commissioner with the Government of India has been made Public Health Commissioner and his deputy has become Director of Medical Research; an Epidemiological Statistical Office, under the Director of Epidemiological Statistics, assisted by expert statisticians, has been created. This central Board advises the Government of India and Provincial Governments on public health matters. The Director of Medical Research co-ordinates the work carried on by the Research Fund Association and the research work carried on under the ægis of the Government of India. The combination of the Public Health and Research Departments is an innovation that is welcomed by all practical sanitarians. The officers of the public health service, finding subjects requiring investigation, call to their aid expert research workers, and when the specific problems are solved will then be in a position to deal with them practically, if the means and power are placed at their disposal. In the various provinces the department presided over by the Sanitary Commissioner is now called Department of Public Health; the Sanitary Commissioner in each province has become the Director of Public Health, and the Deputy Sanitary Commissioners have become Assistant Directors of Public Health. Other changes lately introduced by the Imperial Government are: decentralization of control, opening out the field of recruitment by admission of qualified Indians of proved sanitary talent, and increasing the public health staff; eight more assistant directors of public health have been added and distributed among the Provincial Governments; local governments may select their own director of public health from officers in their public health service, and there is now no limitation of tenure of office of these directors. Selection of assistant directors of public health now also rests with local governments from their own sanitary service; the only conditions laid down by the Imperial Government are that the officer selected must hold a British diploma in public health, a registrable medical qualification, and be an accepted candidate for the public health department. When the local government has no candidate available who is qualified and on its accepted list of candidates the Government of India must be asked for an officer.

The recent reorganization provides for the appointment of a health officer of the first class to the larger municipalities and of the second class for smaller towns; those of the first class must have a registrable medical qualification and a British diploma in public health. The Government of India recognized the weakness in the sanitary education in the Indian universities, and for the present restricts appointments as health officers for the larger towns to D.P.H.s of the United Kingdom. "The necessity for a British diploma in public health will, however, be only temporary, as the Government of India trust that it may be possible to remove the second restriction as soon as arrangements can be made in India which will enable Indians trained in that country to become health officers of the first class. Second-class health officers are required to have had a good general education supplemented by a course of training in public health approved by the local governments. The Government of India left it to local governments to decide in the case of both classes of health officers whether a provincial service should be constituted, or whether the appointments should be made only on conditions which will ensure that qualified men are appointed and that they will have reasonable security of tenure." The Government of India in the same order considered that a service of trained sanitary inspectors should be organized in municipalities based on such standard of population, income, or area as commends itself to the local governments.

It would be advantageous to the larger towns, at least to the capital towns of provinces, to have D.P.H.s who were trained in the United Kingdom as their health officers for some years to come. The emoluments should be high, but private practice should not be allowed. This would prove an excellent training ground for future assistant directors of public health. Municipal bodies appear to prefer health officers of their own selection, officers who would identify themselves with the towns, take special interest in them, help to educate the people in elementary sanitation, and are not liable to be moved about as they would be if attached to an Imperial or Provincial Public Health Department. With this I have some sympathy. The health officer who is looked on as a bird of passage, and one who has no permanent interest in a town, is not likely to meet with the whole-hearted support of the town councillors. The Presidency towns of Calcutta, Bombay, and Madras have had their own health officers for many years. I do not see any insuperable difficulty in enrolling health officers of municipalities in the provincial public health service, so long as it is fully recognized that they are entirely under the municipalities, provided his interests are safeguarded; it seems only reasonable that local governments should give a guarantee of security of tenure just as they should have the power to object to an unsuitable candidate.

The Madras Government has definitely provincialized all health officers; the latter are now only lent to local bodies and municipalities, and I understand that the deputy directors of public health are to be selected from these health officers. This is an important step in the right direction and one that will tend to popularize work in the Public Health Department. It is earnestly hoped that this good example will be followed by all Provincial Governments. The best class of suitable men will be reluctant to take employment entirely under local boards and municipalities in which they would feel an insecurity of tenure of their office.

Young candidates selected for the Public Health Department in provinces should put in an apprenticeship of three months with the health officer of a large town and three months with an assistant director of public health. If the means of providing a sound theoretical and practical training in public health are developed in the various medical colleges there are many reasons for encouraging Indians wholly educated in India to become assistant directors of public health after they have acted as health officers to large municipalities for a certain number of years. A native of India, being intimately acquainted with native social customs and religious prejudices, when he has acquired the confidence of the community with which he works can do a great deal to improve the sanitation of the areas.

Natives of India should be able to obtain a diploma in public health and full instruction in tropical hygiene without having to go to the United Kingdom for them. This is of paramount importance and has been referred to under Medical Education in India. It is easy to formulate the standard of examination for such a diploma ; this has been done in some of the Indian universities already, but it requires a better organization than that which exists to give such a sound practical training as will make medical graduates into useful health officers. I gave very special attention to the question of facilities for training in practical and theoretical hygiene in the five universities (Calcutta, Madras, Bombay, Lucknow, and Lahore), and so far as I could see in none of them could a young man get anything like a useful and practical familiarity with the work he would be called upon to do as a health officer. This is a very serious matter that could so readily be attended to that one is astonished that it has not been seen to years ago. A committee of say three senior specialists in public health could without any difficulty, after going over the public health laboratories of the Indian university colleges, formulate courses of instruction and give details as to the sanitary appliances and equipment required, including models for teaching such rudiments of sanitary engineering as are called for ; the equipment and appliances should be on modern lines.

The Calcutta University grants a diploma in Public Health, but very few have qualified for it up to date ; the Bombay University grants the degrees of Bachelor and Doctor of Public Health, and the Madras University a licence in Sanitary Science. The standards laid down are high, but the facilities to educate up to those standards do not exist; the examination is to a large extent theoretical. The Bombay Government do not select their deputy sanitary commissioners from these, preferring men with a D.P.H. obtained in the United Kingdom; they appoint them, however, as health officers of the first and second class to towns and municipalities. The same rules, I believe, are observed by other local governments. The Imperial Government have not up to date accepted Indian public health diplomas as qualifying for the Public Health Department, and in this they are exercising a wise discretion. For officers not belonging to the I.M.S., a period of two years' probation should be insisted on before they are given posts as assistant directors of public health, local governments having the power in the case of specially selected and qualified candidates to dispense with this probation period.

It is likewise essential that at least one school should be organized, equipped, and staffed in each province for the education and training of sanitary inspectors for employment in municipalities. This is a fundamental necessity, and so very important and at the same time so simple a matter that it is surprising that it has not been undertaken long ago. It should be a permanent institution. One assistant director of public health with a small staff of subordinate teachers, a house with a compound containing models of sanitary appliances, laboratory for elementary analyses, and other equipment for teaching the duties of sanitary inspector, is all that is required. The school should be in a provincial or divisional headquarters town and the local health officer should give demonstrations in the outdoor duties of sanitary inspectors. I believe the late Dr. Turner, C.I.E., when Health Officer of Bombay, trained classes of sanitary inspectors on these lines.

Hitherto the Public Health Department has been unpopular with I.M.S. officers, and the candidates few. Those engaged as assistant directors of public health desire to get civil surgeoncies. The main causes of this unpopularity are the comparatively poor prospects in the department, loss of touch with general professional work, the vast amount of touring to be done, the wide areas to be supervised, and the absence of executive powers. The areas served by assistant directors of public health range from 25,850 square miles in Madras Presidency to 24,597 square miles in Bombay Presidency, and the population from about nine millions in Madras to three and a half millions in Bombay.

At present assistant directors of public health spend much of their time in inspections which have often to be scampered through (unless their tour is made with some special object in view), and in dealing with minor sanitary matters, which in the United Kingdom would be handled by subordinate officials, such as sanitary inspectors and inspectors of nuisances. They have little time to study the various larger sanitary problems of their districts in detail or deal in a scientific way with the different questions connected with the prevention of disease. The result is that there is much uninteresting drudgery, and no scope for genuine ability; these officers lose their early keenness and enthusiasm and finally relinquish sanitary work. The unpopularity of the Public Health Department among I.M.S. officers was one of the factors necessitating recruitment outside that service; many of the posts have now been filled by men not in the I.M.S., mostly Indians.

The insufficient staff of assistant directors of public health and health officers is a defect that requires to be remedied. The Government of India is, I believe, doing all that it can as regards the former. The presidency towns and some of the large provincial towns have, as already stated, their health officers, but the civil surgeon has hitherto been the only health officer of the capital towns of the district. He cannot with all his other duties give the headquarters town a due share of attention; the most he can do is to inspect it occasionally and report on it perfunctorily. Sanitation is still far from efficient once we leave the large towns. The conservancy and drainage are neglected, the water-supply is defective, animals and man are housed together, and in scores of ways the first principles of healthy living are violated.

Large sums of money are being spent on education as compared with what is allotted to medical purposes in India; one is tempted to ask whether it is not an unwise economy that stints expenditure on measures connected with the health and vitality of the vast community of that country. One could mention a few subjects which open extensive fields for preventive measures—malaria and intestinal parasitic diseases, tuberculosis and high infantile mortality, and the care of lying-in women. Much has been done in connexion with malaria, but a great deal remains to be carried out; something has been done to prevent the spread of tuberculosis, but it might be said that so far only the fringe has been touched; the high death-rate of infants clamours for reduction, the deaths and lingering illnesses among women resulting from "dirty midwifery" and the barbarous methods adopted during parturition are tragedies that call for eradication and should arouse profound practical sympathy.

It is curious to witness the unparalleled apathy with which the Indian accepts visitations of cholera, small-pox, relapsing fever, and other epidemics. Malaria, which is responsible for more sickness than all other diseases put together, he calmly looks upon as one of the conditions of his existence. Millions of people died in India from the influenza epidemic of 1918, yet it did not appear to disturb them or their daily life. The only disease that appears to frighten them into activity is plague; one has seen whole villages and bazaars almost deserted a few days after its appearance. This apathy forms one of the fundamental impediments to sanitary improvement in India, especially in rural districts.

The education of the illiterate indigent classes of India in hygiene will take a long time, but it will take longer still to remove their prejudices and cause them to appreciate the advantages such education confers. It is no exaggeration to state that in this matter of knowledge of domestic and general hygiene the poorer classes in rural areas are but little better off than they were a century ago. Poverty, which includes badly constructed and insanitary huts or houses and defective feeding, adds to the difficulties. Teach the people the first principles of domestic and general hygiene is an obvious precept extremely difficult to carry out in the vast continent of India, in which the people have their own ideas of hygiene, some of which are associated with religious ritual and spiritual authority. Our duty, however, is to continue this elementary teaching persistently, combining it with wise and judicious action ; the full benefits of this instruction will not be seen until it becomes part and parcel of the routine life of the people ; we should not be discouraged by slow progress.

Western sanitation is an importation. It is scarcely sixty years old in India and, I believe, would vanish in a single generation or so if not animated and fostered by Western impulse. It has not yet been grafted into the routine life of the people. Education in sanitary matters is only just being generalized ; it certainly is not a subject that is taught universally. As health officer of a large municipal town for ten years I was constantly reminded by fellow municipal commissioners that my recommendations were far too advanced for local application or adoption. The apathy of district boards and town municipalities in sanitary matters is a dead weight which the health officer has to accustom himself to carry in the progress of the race of sanitary improvement. The Municipal Acts of all provinces give comprehensive powers, but most of them are dead letters because of the listless indifference of municipal councillors, most of whom are not educated to even elementary standards in sanitation. I do not include the capital towns of provinces in these remarks ; in the large towns there is a refreshing sanitary awakening, and highly praiseworthy public health work is being done.

The method employed for the registration of vital statistics both in urban and rural areas and the manner in which the results obtained are collected and tabulated are defective in various ways. Statistics supplied by rural areas are very inaccurate and will remain so until better-qualified registrars of births and deaths are employed throughout the country. When health officer of a large municipality in the Deccan, I employed sub-assistant surgeons in this work and obtained fairly reliable records; something of this kind might be tried in rural areas, if the required number of sub-assistant surgeons are available, beginning by their supervising the registration rather than by making them into the actual registrars. There should be no difficulty in such towns as have a health officer with sub-assistant surgeons at the various town dispensaries. We know that the right persons to register births and deaths are medical men, but it is an idle dream to expect anything so complete in India at present. Even in the larger towns and municipalities the vital statistics are not altogether accurate. The registrars, not being medical men, do not possess the knowledge of diseases necessary to classify the death statistics, and the figures furnished by such an agency are necessarily defective.

"There is no organized health staff for more than 90 per cent. of the population; only an insignificant percentage of the people who die annually are seen at any stage of their final illness by persons possessing any sort of medical qualification; the actual recording of vital statistics nearly everywhere in rural India is in the hands of a staff who may have some claim to literacy, but certainly no other qualification. Unless the fallacies are kept carefully in mind, one is tempted to draw more deductions from the vital statistics of India than the figures warrant. Our knowledge of the causes of morbidity and mortality is still woefully deficient."[1] The recorded births and deaths are near the truth, but as to the cause of death much is

[1] *Report of the Sanitary Commissioner with the Government of India*, 1919.

left to speculation. Improvements in the methods of collecting vital statistics must necessarily precede or at least accompany any radical progress in the general health of the community; data regarding the extent of prevalence of preventable disease is fundamental to the putting into operation of organized measures of prevention. The development of a rural health organization commensurate with the importance of the issues involved is the only way of effecting this pressing reform. The health problems of India are of enormous difficulty, perhaps no other part of the civilized world presents health problems of similar magnitude; but a marked improvement in the present state of affairs is possible, provided the money can be found.

The policy should be one of continuous sanitary improvement; the order of the importance of all improvements necessary should be worked out for every town, district, and province, and as far as practicable adhered to. Modifications in the details may be necessary in the future and a revision of the programme is advisable periodically, say every five years or so. This is not a counsel of perfection: it is sound practical sanitary policy, deviation from which has been the cause of much retardation of progress; the general principles upon which sanitary work and progress are based do not change.

The preventive measures adopted by us have not always been wise or judicious, or even efficient. Take the case of epidemic plague, which has now continued in India for over a quarter of a century. In the early days of 1896–1900, when we knew little about the disease, we attempted to eradicate it by such futile measures as segregation, surveillance, and disinfection of the infected, evacuation of the area, all of which except the last-named proved of no avail and met with vigorous resentment and opposition. Evacuation was, as a matter of fact, often adopted spontaneously by the people themselves. Then came inoculation and rat-killing. As we know, inoculation is very useful, but it has its limitations—its protective effects are only temporary, and the immunity conferred is neither complete nor certain. The people resented it bitterly at first, but have now become accustomed to it, and one has had thousands of them coming to the cantonment hospitals clamouring for it.

The path of the sanitary reformer in India is not smooth and easy-going; it is beset with difficulties on all sides, the chief of which are the prejudices, conservatism, dislike of innovations, acceptance of *kismet*, want of education, and entire ignorance of the most rudimentary rules of hygiene on the part of the people. It is a platitude to remark that no preventive measures will succeed in the absence of co-operation of the people. Hindus have actually been seen opening traps containing plague rats and setting free the captures and even sweeping up the bait set for the rats, for among certain sects it is against their principles to take life.

The rate of our economic, industrial, and even social progress in India will to a material extent depend upon the measure of success resulting from well-laid sanitary schemes and measures for the freeing of the people from parasitic infections, including malaria, ankylostomiasis, and ascariasis, which at present militate so seriously against efficiency. In a lecture given by Major-Gen. G. G. Giffard, C.S.I., I.M.S., on July 26, 1922, he stated that hook-worm disease was very widely prevalent in South India. In the Tinnevelly district he knew from statistics that a hundred per cent. of people were affected, and stated that if steps were not taken to eradicate the disease it would sap their vitality and seriously undermine their capacity for work. Hookworms and round-worms are doing much harm to the industrial and agricultural population of India.

Some of the local governments, especially those of Bengal, the United Provinces, and Madras, have started a hygienic publicity compaign under assistant directors of public health, and a number of specially selected civil sub-assistant surgeons in charge of travelling dispensaries after special training are being deputed to give magic-lantern demonstrations and distribute pamphlets on epidemic diseases.

Notwithstanding the formidable difficulties encountered, there have been great sanitary improvements in India during our occupation of the country. The sanitation of larger towns in particular has received a vast amount of attention—water supplies, drainage, and conservancy have been introduced, and more of these are being added in every province yearly; cholera is losing much of its terrors by the measures now adopted and the large staffs employed in preventing it, and in combating outbreaks when they occur; the same, but to a less marked extent, applies to plague and relapsing fever; travelling dispensaries now peregrinate a large area of the country, compaigns against malaria are in operation periodically, a crusade against tuberculosis has been working in several large towns for some years, and measures to reduce infant mortality have been introduced in many cities and towns. There has been a widespread sanitary awakening in India during the last two or three years, and if the present enthusiasm continues the future is full of promise.

CHAPTER VII

AYURVEDIC AND UNANI SYSTEMS OF MEDICINE IN INDIA

Preliminary Remarks.—No *résumé* of the existing state of the medical profession in India would be complete without giving serious attention to the Oriental systems of medicine so largely practised in that country. They play an important rôle and have done so for many centuries. One-third of the indigenous population are being treated by these systems to-day.

Our system of medicine was foreign to the ideas of the people. It was an exotic which took root, but not very vigorously. It was introduced by us originally for the treatment of those under our control; the extension and circumstances of our administration, and the growth of modern medicine have been such as to render it necessary to provide medical relief for those who solicited it. It was natural that the military service, through which allopathic medicine was taken to India, should widen its influence so as to include within its scope both practice and teaching. This introduction of Western medicine established a radical change; such alterations if made too abruptly do not sink in and become part and parcel of the routine life of the people. Some of the very students to whom we teach modern medicine have been brought up in the midst of the Oriental systems; the change therefore is not a simple matter. The soul of Western medicine is not so transitive as many specious thinkers would have us suppose. It is possible that some generations hence the people of India, if properly nurtured in the modern systems of medical treatment, will come to have the same unquestioning faith in it that Western nations have, but a large part of the population have not got that faith yet.

At the period of our original occupation of India the Oriental systems of medicine held the field ; gradually, under the extension of Western medicine, they tended to decline in favour. The *swadeshi* movement gave them the first fillip in recent times. Attempts have been made, not altogether unsuccessfully, under the Reform Scheme, further to develop these systems, and lately the advocates of non-co-operation have made efforts to prevent the sick and suffering poor from attending our hospitals, and have preached the exclusive use of these indigenous systems of medicine. Hundreds of stories are in circulation in towns and villages as to the marvellous cures effected by Ayurvedic and Unani practitioners, and of the high mortality arising from the butchery practised by our surgeons and the harm done by the medicines administered by our physicians.

Unani and Ayurvedic practitioners in a large number of cases have had the calling handed down to them. Some readers will remember the old Persian story which relates that a *hakim*, accompanied by his apprenticed son, attended a nobleman suffering from pain in the abdomen and diagnosed the condition as colic due to eating thirteen mangoes. Both patient and son were astounded at the *hakim's* insight. On leaving the palace the son inquired how his parent knew about the mangoes ; the father told him that as he entered he had counted the thirteen mango stones that were on the ground outside the door.

I remember a time in Calcutta when over the doors of many houses in College Street one read such legends as "Professor of Piles and Fistula" (*sic*), "Professor of Cataract" (couching), "Professor of Spleen" (massage and fire moxæ) in large letters, the "professors" being the descendants of those who had practised these specialities for generations.

The talents of these practitioners vary within extreme

limits from being illiterate impostors and empirics to persons versed in everything that is known in the Ayurvedic or Unani system, these skilled practitioners often also possessing something more than a smattering of Western medicine.

The practitioner of the Ayurvedic or Hindu system of medicine is in some parts of India called a *kaviraj*, in others a *vaidya* or *baida*. Ayurvedic medicine is practised throughout India, but is specially favoured in Bengal, Madras, Central and Southern India. Those who practise Unani medicine are called *hakims ;* the popularity of this system varies in different parts of the country. In the Punjab a large part of the medical practice is in the hand of *hakims*, and it is largely patronized by the people of Hyderabad (Deccan). It has had much to do with retarding the progress of Western medicine in India. It is not easy for the uninitiated to tell the difference between the skilled *kaviraj* and *hakim* and their mountebank imitators.

Some Indians who qualify as allopaths become renegades to Ayurvedic or Unani medicine ; most of these perverts adhere to the ancient system selected, but a few, after making a competency out of it, revert to Western medicine. It is well known that some of the leaders of pure Ayurvedic practice make considerable fortunes out of their calling, and when consulted in mofussil cases from the larger towns charge heavy fees. I have known one Indian allopathic practitioner who, when ill himself, called in a *kaviraj* to treat him ; and I have known some who meet Ayurvedic or Unani practitioners in consultation regularly, and my experience is not unique. One might here mention incidentally that some medical graduates and diplomates of our Indian universities become homœopathic practitioners, especially in Calcutta, and some have acquired great reputations as such ; but there are likewise a host of irregular homœopathic " doctors " in India, who have had little or no training for the medical profession.

There are Ayurvedic and Unani dispensaries in almost

every city and large town in India. My personal knowledge of these systems was acquired while practising for ten years in Hyderabad (Deccan), where they flourished.

a. Ayurvedic or Hindu System of Medicine

The Ayurveda, or Vedas dealing with medicine, were believed to have been communicated directly from Brahma to Dacsha, the Prajapati his son, who passed them on to the sons of the sun (Surja), who gave them to Indra. Indra is reputed to have taught Bharadwaja, a learned sage; these incidents date back to the primitive age of the priest-physician. This spiritual or inspired origin of the Ayurveda is important. The great works of this system are those of Charaka, Sushruta, Vagbhalta, and Madhava. The *Charaka Samhita* and *Sushruta Samhita* are the venerable works upon which the system is based; these are the supreme authorities of the *kavirajes*. It is highly probable that, as Dr. A. F. R. Hoernle[1] states, both these works in their present form are composite, and that the *Charaka Sushruta* was compiled in the second century A.D., and the *Charaka Samhita* of Dridhabala between the seventh and ninth centuries. A vast amount of surgical procedure and empirical medicine is gathered together in these volumes. The literature of Ayurvedic medicine has remained stationary since the Middle Ages, and any progress made since then has been traditional; indeed progress was impeded by the force of authority under which these books existed, and by isolation of India from advancing science.

A valuable translation of the *Charaka Samhita*[2] was published some years ago and reviewed in the March 1918 issue of the *Indian Medical Gazette*, by the late Lieut.-Col. W. D. Sutherland, C.I.E., I.M.S. The translation must have involved years of arduous labour, and as an historical record of the state of medicine in India a few thousand years ago is most valuable, and we are greatly indebted

[1] *Studies on the Medicine of Ancient India*, Part I.

[2] *Charaka Samhita*, translated into English and published by Avinash Chandra Kaviratna, Parts I and II (Calcutta, 1908).

to the learned *kaviraj* for this work. I would ask the reader's indulgence while I make a few quotations, *literatim et verbatim*, from the translation under reference to give some notion of the principles upon which the Ayurvedic system is based and leave him to draw his own conclusions.

The translator states that the subjects of wind or *vayu*, bile or *pitta*, and phlegm or *kapha* must be properly understood before the Charaka system can be comprehended. "Wind is not the atmosphere, bile is not the secretion of the liver, and phlegm is not the secretions that persons with cold throw out. They are technical terms that imply certain states of the physical constitution." They are forces which act on the body in health and disease. "The hypogastrium or pubic region, the place where the fæces collect, the region about the loins, the thighs, feet and bones are the seats of the wind. That portion of the stomach, however, where digestion goes on, among the seats of the wind is in particular the seat thereof. Sweat, the thorax, saliva, blood and that portion of the stomach where the undigested food remains, are the seats of bile. Amongst these, the last is especially the seat of bile. The thorax, the head, the throat, all the joints, that portion of the stomach which holds the undigested food and the fat, are the seats of phlegm" (*Charaka Samhita*, p. 221).

Some advanced *kavirajes* of to-day declare that "the Sages used the word *vayu*, *pitta*, and *kapha* in a sense distinct from that in which we use the terms wind, bile, and phlegm, because by these terms they signified nervous force, metabolism, phagocytosis and what not." Such sophistry might beguile the laity and puzzle judges and barristers in India, but can carry no weight with us to-day.

Regarding the *pulse* it is stated :

"In the case of male patients the pulse is felt at the wrist of the right hand, and in that of female patients that of the left hand. The pulse of a healthy adult is not uniform all day long. In the morning it appears to be cool ; at midday it seems to be hot ; while in the evening it becomes quicker" (I, p. 20). "Generally, in any disease due to excitement of the wind the pulse is said to assume a curvilinear motion. In any disease due to excitement of the bile the pulse becomes quick. In any disease due to excitement of the phlegm the pulse becomes slow, regular and heavy. The curvilinear motion under excitement of the wind may be like the course of a serpent, a leech, etc. The quickness of the pulse due to the excitement of the bile may be like the motion of a crow, or of the francoline partridge, or of the frog. The slow, regular and heavy pulse which is due to excitement of the phlegm, it is similarly said resembles the motion of the swan, the peacock, the pigeon, the dove, the cock, etc. When fever has set in the pulse becomes hot and quick. In intermittent fevers appearing on alternate days, the pulse is sometimes felt at the root of the thumb and sometimes by its sides" (I, p. 24). On one occasion I earned undeserved merit in an Indian nobleman's family, whose ordinary medical adviser was a celebrated *kaviraj*. I was requested to feel the pulse of a lady who was standing behind a door that was ajar. It appeared to me to be an ordinary healthy pulse, and I casually remarked that I could find nothing wrong with it. A murmur of applause arose in the room beyond the door, and I was told that she was not the patient. It afterwards transpired that during this preliminary stage of the proceedings I was on trial, and that my lucky shot secured me the confidence of the family.

Regarding the *tongue* in disease it is stated:

"If the wind predominates in the constitution the colour of the tongue resembles the leaves of the teak. . . . If the bile predominates the tongue presents a red or darkish hue, while if the phlegm predominates, it becomes thick and white. The prickles over it become confluent and it constantly secretes saliva" (I, 22).

I was once consulted by a family to see an adult Indian lady with an abdominal tumour, alleged to be due to pregnancy: she had previously been attended by an Ayurvedic practitioner. I found her covered with a sheet, and on asking to see her tongue they made a slit in the middle of the sheet (which consisted of two halves sewn lengthwise in the middle) through which the tongue was protruded. The case turned out to be one of malarial enlargement of the spleen, that organ practically filling the whole abdominal cavity. The family considered that I should have been able to diagnose the case by the condition of the tongue.

The following are among the medical philosophical teachings:

> "The physician should not take up that man for treatment who has got dropsical swellings of his feet, whose calves have lost all compactness, and whose thighs have become exceedingly weak. That man should not be treated with medicines whose hands, feet, arms, and abdomen show signs of swelling, who has become divested of complexion, strength and appetite. That man should be forsaken (by the physician) from a distance whose chest is largely filled with phlegm, which is of a blue, or yellow, or of a red colour, and which comes out constantly. The physician possessed of knowledge should forsake from a distance that man the hair on whose body stands erect, whose urine becomes dense, and who has fever with a dry cough and whose flesh has been reduced. The wise are of opinion that the period of life has run short of that man whose spittle and fæces sink in water" (*Charaka Samhita*, p. 991).

The ethics of these philosophical utterances call for no further comment here.

Regarding the prognosis of disease I make the following quotation from another Ayurvedic work: "The favourable or unfavourable termination of a disease may be predicted from the appearance, speech, dress and demeanour of the messenger sent to call a physician, or from the nature of the asterism and the lunar phase marking the time of the arrival, or from the direction of the wind blowing at the time, or from the nature of omens seen by him on the road, or from the posture or speech of the physician himself. A messenger belonging to the same caste as the patient himself should be regarded as an auspicious omen, whereas one from a different caste would indicate a fatal or an unfavourable termination of the disease."[1]

[1] *Sushruta Samhita*, translation by Kaviraj Kunja Lal Bishagratna, p. 270.

There are several published works on the Ayurvedic system of medicine as practised and taught to-day. One of the best known is *The Ayurvedic System of Medicine*, or *An Exposition in English of Hindu Medicine, as occurring in Charaka Sushruta, Bhagata, and other Authoritative Sanskrit Works, Ancient and Modern*, by Kaviraj Nagendra Nath Sen Gupta, 3 vols., Calcutta, revised edition, 1909. This work was also reviewed by the late Lieut.-Col. W. D. Sutherland, C.I.E., I.M.S., in the *Indian Medical Gazette*, February 1919, who threw much light on the subject of Ayurvedic practice of the present day. The object of the author was to place before the English-speaking world, and particularly before physicians and surgeons practising the Western method of medicine, the knowledge which the Rishis had of disease and its cure. This work gives in a condensed form the views propounded in larger works on Hindu medicine.

It is stated in the preface that little or no progress has been made in midwifery since Sushruta's time. The midwifery of Sushruta consisted in the use of incantations to expedite the delivery of the fœtus until its death. "When the fœtus was known to be dead, then, and then only, were the various manipulations described to be employed." The Ayurveds of to-day claim that anatomy as taught by Sushruta was of a very high standard and that the methods of dissection were much better than they are in our present Western medical schools. This is so gross an exaggeration that refutation of it is superfluous. Correspondingly high claims are made in regard to the surgery of the early Hindus. Sushruta's surgery was probably excellent for the time in which he practised, and possibly contrasted favourably with that adopted in other civilized countries, but it has no grounds for comparison with modern surgery; it would now be considered barbaric butchery. It is also claimed that as Ayurvedic methods have undergone no serious change for over 2,000 years they must be perfect. The quotations given show the fallacy of this statement. There is much sophistry and misrepresentation in the comparisons of Ayurvedic with Western medicine. Some writers on modern Ayurvedic treatment scruple at no artifice or exaggeration that in their judgment might depreciate Western medicine.

The most extravagant effects are claimed for the medicines employed in this system and an elaborate Ayurvedic Pharmacopœia is in use. In Kaviraj Nagendra Nath Gupta's work, two large volumes are devoted to the description and effects of Ayurvedic drugs and therapeutic methods. I will quote a single sample: "The poison of black cobra or krait, taken for medicinal purposes, should be first mixed with mustard oil and dried in the sun. It should then be macerated first in the expressed juice of betel leaves, then in the expressed juice of the leaves of *baka* (*Sesbania grandiflora*), and lastly, in decoction of *kura* (*Aplotaxis auriculata*). The process of maceration in each should be repeated three times" (vol. ii, p. 26).

One of the principles of the system is that diseases are the results of the operations of evil spirits who have to be pacified by various offerings and propitiated by incantations. Regarding the diseases of children it is stated that these "are due to the action of certain spirits who were belated in obtaining lucrative posts in the retinue of the Destroyer and were compelled to secure power to tax sorrowing parents, who might have committed any of the hundred-odd ritual faults by afflicting their offspring." One searches in vain for anything approaching definite and rational therapeutics in this system. We have in a *modern* Ayurvedic work a complex combination of drugs extolled as being able to cure such diverse conditions as obesity and gonorrhœa, and another extensive combination alleged to effect a cure in all diseases of women however caused. Throughout the literature we are made conscious of the influence of "authority" and "inspiration" in the teaching handed down.

Another very readable work which deals largely with the Ayurvedic among other systems of treatment is

Review of the History of Medicine, by the late Thomas A. Wise, Bengal Medical Service (W. Thacker, Bombay and Calcutta, 1867); to this excellent treatise I am much indebted.

There are reasons for considering that through the ages the Ayurvedic system of medicine gradually underwent serious deterioration. Under the influence of wars and invasions, new religions were introduced; caste distinctions became more rigid; Brahmins fearing to touch blood or diseased matter left the study of medicine to the lower and illiterate castes; hospitals which had in an earlier era been erected by Buddhists were abandoned, and ancient Hindu medicine sank to a low position; it was in a late stage of decline when the British founded medical schools and hospitals at the end of the eighteenth and first part of the nineteenth centuries.

There are no grounds for comparing the Oriental systems of medicine of the present day with that of modern Western medicine. From the fifteenth century onwards Western medicine has been developing with the aid of physical and biological sciences, anatomy, physiology, chemistry, and pathology. The Unani and Ayurvedic practitioner of old knew nothing of these sciences and he knows but little to-day. With the Ayurvedic system Western medicine has had no relation until comparatively modern times; to-day many of the more advanced Ayurveds practise a hybrid combination of the two.

The Ayurvedic system was the most advanced form of medicine and surgery for centuries after it was instituted; it served its purpose. From what has been stated regarding Ayurvedic practice of medicine, pathology, and therapeutics it may be considered by the unprejudiced Western mind that no modern civilized Government ought to foster any scheme for the advancement of such a system in the practical life of India to-day, and there may be many who feel it to be quite wrong to allot any public funds to encourage either this or the Unani system—that neither time nor money ought to be frittered away in these prehistoric absurdities. As will be seen later on, I am not disposed to assume this attitude of lofty aloofness and antagonism ; I prefer endeavouring to make these systems instruments to serve the people of India in a highly practical way.

b. Unani, Tibbi, or Græco-Arabic System of Medicine

According to Garrison, Arabian medicine began with Nestor, a Christian heretic priest driven by religious persecution from Byzantium to Edessa in Mesopotamia, where he commenced the study of medicine. Pursued here, he fled to Persia and established the Gundeshapur Medical College wherein were trained the first founders of this system. It spread to Arabia, which country in those days attracted many learned people from all parts on account of the reputed wisdom of the Caliphs, and the scientific attainments of the teachers. These visitors brought with them many herbs and drugs which were investigated. The decline of Arabic medicine began in the thirteenth century, with the fall of Cordova in 1236, and the invasion of Baghdad in 1258, when its former scholars were attracted to the school of Salerno.

There are several Arabic works which include dictionaries and translations from the Greek, also original works on general medicine and pharmacopœias. One of the greatest masters was Rhazes of Ray in Iraq-i-Ajam ; he was taught at Baghdad, was the first director of the Ray Hospital, and later of that of Baghdad, A.D. 923. Avicenna, physician to the Sultan of Bukhara, wrote the *Book of the Canon.* Albucassas prepared a medical encyclopædia, chiefly valued for its surgical portion, which was translated into Latin in the twelfth century and for long remained the standard surgery of Europe. Much that is in the Unani system of to-day was practised for hundreds of years in Europe and did not die in that continent until the fourteenth century. Indeed the Unani system is the Græco-Arabic system of Rhazes and Avicenna, which formed the primary foundation of Western medicine ; it was carried to India by the Mahomedan invaders and is now practised by *hakims* over a good part of that country. It was not affected by the advance of science, and such change as has taken place has been adopted from modern medicine within the last century. The Greeks of the time of Hippocrates, and Aristotle practised medicine after their degree of enlightenment; to-day there are no traces of their methods left in Greece; the School of Alexandria, the most advanced of its time, filled its rôle and died out; the same holds good of Salerno.

c. Schools of Oriental Systems of Medicine in India

The question may be asked, what part have we taken in India in connexion with the Ayurvedic and Unani medicine? The reply entails a brief review of the education in the Oriental systems adopted during the last century.

In 1827 classes were opened in Calcutta almost simultaneously in the Sanskrit College for teaching the Ayurvedic system and at the Madrassah (Mahomedan College) for the Unani system. These, it would seem, were under the H.E.I.C. and did not prove to be satisfactory. "The system of Galen and Hippocrates and of the Shasters, with the addition of a few scraps of science, was taught in classes which had been attached for the purpose to the Arabic and Sanskrit College at Calcutta, the object of which was to train up 'native doctors' or assistants to the European medical officers. There was only one teacher attached to this institution and he delivered his lectures in Hindustani. The only books open to the pupils were a few short tracts which had been translated for their use into that language; the only dissection practised was that of the inferior animals."[1] Various half-hearted efforts were made at different times during the last sixty years to resuscitate the teaching of the ancient systems, and their schools have slowly developed.

[1] Sir E. C. Trevelyan, *On the Education of the People of India*, p. 27.

At the present time there are several Ayurvedic medical schools in India, such as the Hindu Medical College in Calcutta. The course there is for five years; the pupils are mostly sons of *kavirajes*; they are from seventeen to twenty years of age. Anatomy is taught by animal dissection; the teaching is in Bengali, the pupils are trained to compound indigenous medicines; there is a collection of drugs for instructional demonstration, a small botanic garden, and a library.

There is a large Unani school in Delhi which is at present flourishing. Several other smaller schools exist in various parts of India (as will be seen in the context) for training Ayurvedic and Unani practitioners.

The Punjab University subsidizes the teaching of Ayurvedic and Unani medicine. In former years the teaching was under the ægis of that University in connexion with the Oriental College, Lahore, and anatomy was taught the pupils at the Lahore Medical College. Then the Ayurvedic classes were transferred to the Dayanand Anglo-Vedic College, and the Unani classes to the Islamia College in 1898–99; the University makes small grants for their maintenance provided that the staff employed are approved by the University. Definite curricula are gone through, usually lasting two years. The arrangements regarding clinical teaching are not satisfactory. A review of the curriculum indicates that the course of instruction is a modification of the Western medical curriculum. The official report states that "books dealing with pathology, pharmacy, materia medica, anatomy, physiology, midwifery, chemistry, and physics were taught, and that besides arrangements for practical work in the College, a charitable dispensary was started in a hired building to give further practical training to the students. The dispensary had, however, to be closed after a few months." At the Unani classes at the Islamia College there were 65 students on the roll with an average attendance of 52. The students include not only Mahomedans but also Hindus and Sikhs. In April 1917, 41 students appeared at the *hakim* examination, of whom 21 were successful.[1]

The Standing Committee of the All-India Ayurvedic and Unani Tibbi Conference addressed to the Government of India several resolutions on March 15, 1918, the following, *inter alia*: "That Government should be pleased to take steps to improve the ancient systems of medicine and to place them on a scientific basis." The Reception Committee of the All-India Mahomedan Education Conference about the same time submitted the following resolution: "That this Conference urges upon the Government of India the desirability of reviewing and popularizing the Unani System of Medical Education which has been so useful in dealing with tropical diseases, and of establishing Unani Medical Colleges at least in the Presidency towns."

One distinguished Indian[2] in his evidence before the Calcutta University Commission stated: "The University should not ignore the claims of indigenous systems of medicine prevalent in the country. The University should do something to stimulate the proper study of the literature on these subjects under duly recognized masters. There is much scope for study, improvement, and research in these directions." Another Indian[3] before the same Commission recommended special Government grants for the establishment and maintenance of Ayurvedic colleges and suggested that Ayurvedic medicine should be under the ægis of the Calcutta University. Sir G. Dass Banerjee suggested that the active principles and modes of action of remedies which have stood the test of experience for centuries require investigation by scientific methods, and that the study of the system should be

[1] *Annual Report of the Punjab University for* 1917, quoted by *Calcutta University Commission Report*, vol. iii, Part I, p. 60. I am indebted to this latter report for much of my information on Ayurvedic and Unani education.

[2] Mr. M. Banerjee, Lecturer on Experimental Psychology, University College of Science, Calcutta.

[3] Rai M. C. Mitra, Bahdr.

encouraged by the University. Another witness suggested that the University of Calcutta should confer doctors' degrees in Ayurvedic medicine.

In the warm discussion that preceded the formation of the committee of inquiry into the Oriental system in Madras in November 1921 (*vide infra*) one of the Indian members of the council stated that "it was a quite unwarranted thing to look down on the Ayurvedic system of medicine. The Ayurvedic system was just as scientific as the Western system of medicine. It was being availed of by the masses all over the country. The medical aid provided by Government to taxpayers was totally inadequate. In cases of snake-bite and rabies the Western system failed while the Eastern system succeeded."

The working of the Montagu-Chelmsford Reform Scheme has given a forcible forward push to the Unani and Ayurvedic systems. The Medical Services Committee of 1919 fully anticipated that this would be the case. In their report they stated: "These systems, the Ayurvedic and Unani, Hindu and Arabic, still appeal to the masses, in a less degree to the educated. The records of the debates in various Legislative Councils on the subject of registration of medical practitioners show this clearly; it is probable that when Provincial Governments become in some degree dependent on popular votes they will be frequently urged to spend public money on Ayurvedic and Unani schools and dispensaries. On the other hand, all available funds are badly needed for extending medical relief and sanitary prevention on Western lines. . . . We are convinced that unless vigorously supported and pioneered by thoroughly efficient and energetic Government service, Western medicine and methods of sanitation will rather lose than gain ground in this country (India)." The Medical Services Committee thrashed out this matter; we felt instinctively that as soon as the Reforms Scheme came into operation clamours for the allotment of funds to those systems would crop up, and that these allotments would be made at the expense of Western medicine. During the last year the Bihar and Orissa Government had before it a proposal to allot from the medical budget large sums for the encouragement of Ayurvedic practice, but that Government declined to do so. The Madras Legislative Council have recently had a contretemps over the same thing, but likewise refused to divert funds for this purpose. The question was dealt with last year by the Indian National Congress when it was claimed that Ayurvedic medicine was " just as scientific as modern allopathic medicine." In 1920 the Imperial Government expressed sympathy with the Oriental systems of medicine and made a grant to the Unani Tibbi Medical School at Delhi.

The subject of the indigenous systems of medicine was again introduced and discussed in the Indian Council of State in February 1921, a resolution being proposed that the Government of India should recommend to every provincial government the desirability of having an Ayurvedic medical college, of taking measures to develop indigenous drugs, and appointing *vaidyas* and *hakims* in every dispensary to treat patients by indigenous methods. An account of the debate was sent to provincial governments, but the Government of India did not accept the proposal contained in the resolution as the matter was not one for it to deal with.

" It was evident from the discussion that some of the Indian members have a belief in the efficacy of the indigenous systems, but it was urged on the other hand that these systems had made no advance for centuries and was hopelessly below modern standards." [1] There is the probability that the provincial governments are likely to take their cue from the views of the Imperial Government.

These debates and resolutions in the Imperial Council Chamber and the various Provincial Legislative Assemblies, and those in the National Congress, indicate that Western medicine has not got as firm a hold on the people of India as many of us have believed ; it is still, in a sense, competing for popularity with the Oriental systems which are to

[1] *The Pioneer Mail,* March 1921.

a large extent favoured by the people who adhere to the faith of their ancestors.

I am of opinion that for the present the universities of India should not undertake the training of students in the Ayurvedic and Unani systems. These systems have neglected to adapt themselves to the progress which sciences have imposed on Western medicine during the last three or four hundred years. In a speech made by Sir Sankaran Nair at the Ayurvedic and Unani Tibbi College at Delhi, March 24, 1918, he stated to the students: "The study of modern sciences is indispensable for medicine." His Excellency Lord Pentland, Governor of Madras, in February 1918, in opening the Ayurvedic Hospital in the Cochin State, said: "Medicine, whether it be called Ayurvedic, Unani, or Western, must follow the same methods and the same aims and submit to the same tests; any system of medicine must be correlated with every advance in the allied sciences such as chemistry and physiology." He emphasized also the necessity for qualifying examinations and standards.

d. Practical Remarks on the Oriental Systems of Medicine in India

The Medical Registration Act of India came into operation in 1916. An unqualified medical man can now no longer call himself doctor. It was framed to defeat the unqualified practitioner of Western medicine and the men granted diplomas by unauthorized medical schools, and to prevent such men practising allopathy. This Act excludes the practitioners of Oriental systems—it does not interfere with the *kaviraj* and *hakim*; they remain, learned and quack alike, uncontrolled. It will have been seen that the practice of the Ayurved is associated with religious ritual and observance, and that any legislation undertaken to regulate it should call for much thought, sympathy, and delicate handling. I believe it would be wise for provincial governments to take a census of all *kavirajes* and *hakims*, as well as of the different classes of mountebanks that mimic them. I would also suggest that a full inquiry be made as to the methods by which they go through their training or acquire proficiency in their calling. Personally I consider that there would be no difficulty in getting together two small selected committees, one of allopaths and Ayurveds, and another of allopaths and Unanis, to formulate curricula of education. Would it not be a protection to the people to prescribe, with the co-operation of the leaders of these systems, a course of theoretical and practical training extending over some years, and laying down the scope of examinations to be passed before granting a qualification to practise? Might it not be possible gradually to introduce the essentials of modern science into the educational processes and thus eventually graft rational principles on to what is at present nebulous, vague, empiric, and inefficient? There are many who share my opinion that it is possible to convert these Oriental systems into instruments for conferring vast benefits on the people of India by showing some sympathy with them, so that they may in an improved form be able to reach the poorer classes in the more remote villages and districts, where, for many years to come, we cannot hope to place Western medicine within their reach. This will take many years of persistent effort, and no immediate good results can be expected. Personally I can visualize practitioners of these systems converted into a large army of native doctors affording an enormous amount of medical relief on a combined Western and Oriental system, the latter having eliminated from it whatever is pernicious. I can see no other way in which adequate medical treatment will reach the whole of the masses for the next hundred years.

This, as a matter of fact, appears to be the direction in which opinion in the last few years appears to be leaning. Sir William Edwards, Dir.-Gen. I.M.S., in the Council of State quite lately reminded his audience that there was strictly speaking no such thing as Eastern medicine or Western medicine; that India was the only country in which the ancient system of medicine had survived, while China and Japan had adopted the modern medicine in vogue in the rest of the civilized world. The proper course therefore was to absorb into modern practice the features of Ayurvedic and Unani medicine which had been proved by scientific research to be of real value. This the Government of India has declared itself to be already trying to accomplish.

In a Press notice issued by the United Provinces Government in October 1921 it is stated: "The Ayurvedic and Unani systems of medicine are still widely popular in this province. The policy of government is to help in the extension to the poor of all kinds of medical relief, including indigenous systems of medicine, and for encouragement of the latter they have included a sum of Rs. 25,000 in the current year's budget. The following were considered the best ways of distributing this money:

"1. To give grants to local bodies to establish travelling or stationary Ayurvedic or Unani dispensaries;

2. To give grants to existing Ayurvedic or Unani dispensaries provided they are controlled by influential managing committees;

3. To give grants to existing institutions for the training of *vaids* or *hakims* subject to the same proviso." [1]

The U.P. Government also sanctioned an allotment of Rs. 50,000 for an Ayurvedic College established at Hardwar.

A committee was appointed in November 1921 in Madras to inquire into the Ayurvedic and Unani systems as practised in that Presidency. In January 1922 the committee began preparing a list of the Ayurvedic and Unani institutions in the Madras Presidency, including those of indoor and outdoor patients, teaching institutions, and institutions for special diseases like leprosy and tuberculosis, and a list of practitioners in the Madras Presidency following or proficient in the Ayurvedic and Unani systems with their qualifications, noting to what extent these were trained in Western medicine. This committee is also

[1] *The Pioneer Mail*, October 21, 1921.

collecting evidence from the leading practitioners who are specially qualified in both indigenous and Western systems. This is the first inquiry of the kind carried out in India, and will, I believe, be fruitful in giving us unbiased scientific criticism on these systems. The leading practitioners of these systems are also giving evidence in this inquiry and the committee are likewise inspecting hospitals, dispensaries, colleges, schools, museums, libraries, botanical gardens and the like where experiments are already in progress in the matter of affording medical relief and medical education on the basis of indigenous systems of medicine. The work of this committee will be of inestimable value in assisting the Imperial and Provincial Governments to formulate a scheme along the lines of which the indigenous systems may be safely encouraged and recognized by the State.[1]

From the many debates that took place in the Imperial Legislative Council and provincial councils in connexion with the Ayurvedic and Unani systems it was obvious that many members believed in the beneficial effects of the drugs employed in them. These advocates expressed the opinions that drugs used were as efficacious as those in the B.P., that the indigenous systems were much more economical than Western medicine, and that a careful investigation would discover a large number of very valuable but hitherto unknown remedies.

After these discussions in the various councils the Madras Government appointed Dr. M. C. Koman, an Indian medical man attached to the Medical College, Madras, to carry out an investigation. During two years, while so employed, he submitted three reports. He visited a large number of Ayurvedic pharmacies and dispensaries and collected the most important drugs and preparations, and experimented with these on suitable patients in the wards of the Madras General Hospital. His investigations were limited to the therapeutic actions of these drugs and compounds ; with the means at his disposal he was unable

[1] *The Lancet*, January 14, 1922, p. 95.

to carry out more ambitious inquiries. He states that the work of Ainslie (1826), Warden and Hooper, Waring, W. C. Dutt, K. L. Dey and others, and the reports of the Indigenous Drugs Committee, prove that all important indigenous medicinal plants have already been investigated, and remarks: "In vain have I attempted to find any drug whose reputed marvellous properties are shrouded in mystery or have not been already known." With few exceptions he found the *vaidyas* and *hakims* generally unversed and unintelligent, though industrious and well-meaning, and nearly all evinced a firm conviction and belief in the intervention of evil spirits and offered many curious and absurd rules for averting their machinations.[1] An important point elicited by Dr. Koman was that the cost of maintaining an Ayurvedic dispensary is much the same as that of one of our own dispensaries, whilst the Ayurvedic dispensary limits its work to medical treatment except in the case of couching for cataract.

He found a few drugs of real value, but advised that much more work should be done on them before they can be universally recommended. He advised that all the Ayurvedic and Unani drugs found efficacious should be included in the lectures on materia medica and pharmacology in the medical colleges and schools.

Included in Dr. Koman's list are: (1) *Hydnocarpus inebrians*, a potent drug in ameliorating the complications of leprosy; (2) Kirmani (*Artemisia maritima*, a substitute for santonin; (3) Chempullanhi (*Colycopterus floribunda*) an efficacious anthelmintic; (4) *Boerhavia diffusa*, a good diuretic in cases of anasarca, the result of Bright's disease.

In the second appendix is given a list of forty drugs or compounds found to be useful, but not so effective as medicines already in the B.P.; they are cheaper and more easily obtained than their B.P. equivalents.[2] the Government of Madras ordered that these experiments be con-

[1] *The Lancet*, July 2, 1921, p. 40.
[2] *The Lancet*, July 2, 1921, pp. 39, 40.

tinued with the view to eventually incorporating the useful drugs in the Pharmacopœia of the Madras Presidency.

The account of the actions taken by the Madras Government afforded me profound personal satisfaction; it is on the lines detailed that we shall eventually remove the cloud of mystery in which the Ayurvedic and Unani systems of medicine have been enveloped and that we shall eventually know the truth in connexion with these systems. The Madras Government under the able administrative medical guidance of Major-General G. G. Giffard, C.S.I., I.M.S., is taking a leading part in this and other large medical questions. Personally I am disposed to consider that Ayurvedic and Unani drugs and curative methods demand a much more comprehensive investigation than that to which Dr. Koman was limited, and that the work should be in the hands of a more or less permanent committee consisting of a chemist, pharmacologist, an Ayurvedic and a Unani practitioner of high repute, and a physiologist, who should be provided with all that is necessary to conduct their work under the best possible modern scientific conditions; they should be able to co-opt a botanist when one was required. This work will take some years, but the various questions will then be solved once for all. Such a committee it is presumed would either take the place of the Indigenous Drugs Committee, or the latter could be reconstituted to take on this new rôle. I doubt whether sufficient data have been collected as yet to arrive at a complete scientific opinion on this subject, and should be disposed to deprecate any expression of opinion until all the data that can possibly be obtained are on the record, and have been thoroughly digested and deliberated on.

I feel that our attitude of indifference and hostility has hitherto not been altogether wise; it has generated much sympathy on the part of many of the people in favour of the *kaviraj* and *hakim*, whom they look upon as being down-trodden and repressed. It has likewise tended to the creation of a harmful class of quack and charlatan, who profess to practise these Oriental systems without any knowledge whatever of them. A cursory glance at the advertisements of the vernacular periodicals, and journals in English managed by Indians, will show how the unfortunate public is being victimized by these irregular practitioners.

There is little doubt but that these Oriental systems do a certain amount of good among the people, partly arising from their faith in them. Were the *kaviraj* or *vaid* and *hakim* to do harm and afford no relief, their systems would not have acquired the confidence they enjoy at present; the Hindu system could not have survived for over 2,000 years, nor the Arabic system many centuries, if they did nothing but harm. I entertain doubts as to the political wisdom of ignoring the hold these Oriental systems have on the people, and I am quite sure that adopting an attitude of contempt is not the way to meet them.

I have already adverted to the part that lectureships on pharmacology and on the history of medicine in our Indian universities could play in diffusing a knowledge of Ayurvedic and Unani medicine, and to the desirability of our absorbing any part of those systems, traditional or recorded, that are found to be of service in the relief of human suffering and the cure of disease.

From all one has seen and heard during the last few years of one's service in India there seemed to be a desire on the part of Ayurvedic and Unani practitioners to bring their systems into more intimate relation with modern scientific medicine, and I feel strongly that this spirit should be in every way encouraged. It is highly probable that with greater sympathy from us we shall ourselves benefit by acquiring the useful parts of their knowledge. Indeed, if such a policy is adopted, and carried out steadily for a few generations, a time may come when the Oriental systems of medicine practised in India will merge into the Western, and finally the differences between them vanish. This is an ambitious programme, but I feel that it is the ideal we should aim at.

It would be possible to organize the issue of propaganda in favour of modern medicine, comparing modern with ancient methods, and bringing the advantages of the former home to the people through the press, by placards, notices, lectures, pictorial displays, cinemas, etc. One is not disposed to advocate such a course. If Western medicine and surgery, as practised by allopaths in India, is not able to stand on its own merits, it will in course of time cease to be practised. On the other hand, Ayurvedic medicine has lived over 2,000 years in India, and like a certain brand of whisky it is "still going strong"; and unless something conspicuously better is introduced and maintained among the many millions who favour it, there is every possibility of its vitality increasing.

Western medicine is advancing and growing in popularity in the larger towns and centres of population where it is extensively practised. Its progress is very tardy in villages and outlying districts in which Ayurvedic and Unani medicine still claim millions of votaries among the masses of the people. We have been educating the people to the use of the Western system of medicine; wherever that system has had a fair chance they have got to prefer it; and on the whole the circle embracing it has until quite recently been widening yearly. The system of modern medicine will not only hold its own, but will absorb and drive out all others if it is freely brought within the reach of the people. It has been one of our great privileges to take the blessings of Western medicine to India; it has reached a certain stage of development there. Should we stop at this stage? Extend the benefits of Western medicine to the utmost possible limits; the results will appeal to the people more strongly than any other form of advocacy. How can we expect them to abandon their own systems in which they have faith if we do not substitute something better in its place? The inference is that a larger number of medical men and more hospitals are called for, especially in those areas not yet touched by Western methods.

It would be most lamentable for the people of India were these ancient systems—as now practised—to acquire any serious degree of ascendancy over modern medicine; were this to happen it would take many generations to regain the comparatively favourable position Western medicine holds in the country to-day.

CHAPTER VIII

MEDICAL WORK OF WOMEN IN INDIA

1. Women Doctors

There is a progressively increasing tendency for the women of India to take up medicine as a profession. The work of training women doctors grew very slowly until about ten years ago, when it seemed to make a forward leap. Among the earlier beginnings were those of the Medical School, Hyderabad (Deccan), about 35 years ago, where I lectured for 10 years. We had an average of 10 women and girl students, several of whom subsequently qualified in the United Kingdom. At the present time there are women pupils in all the medical colleges and medical schools in India. The Lady Hardinge Medical College, which is exclusively for the education of women doctors, accommodates 60 pupils, of whom 30 are Anglo-Indians, 5 Europeans, and 25 Indians; most of them read and work for the M.B., B.S., of the Lahore University. After qualifying many of the women of the various colleges take up work as house physicians and house surgeons in different women's hospitals. Subsequently they are placed in independent charge of small hospitals, but some go to the U.K. to complete their education and take home degrees, although this is not necessary for the Women's Medical Service. Women students come off very well as compared with male students in their training in Midwifery and diseases of women and children in India—there is no let or hindrance to them as there is to male pupils, with the result that after finishing their five years' curriculum each one has had almost expert training in midwifery and diseases of women. Applications for admission into the Lady Hardinge Medical College are much in excess of the vacancies.

It is satisfactory to find that there is at the present time a large demand for women doctors throughout India, chiefly from public bodies such as municipalities and district boards. The supply of women doctors to meet these is insufficient. The conditions of service under these bodies are, however, unsatisfactory in many ways, and the hospitals in which women doctors have to work call for improvement both as to structure and equipment. These defects can be remedied without much difficulty; the main point is that the demand for women doctors has arisen. It appears to me that it would be much more satisfactory to form a separate medical service for women in each province, working under the local Government, the postings, transfers, promotion, etc., being under that Government. What women doctors appear to apprehend at present is that in serving local municipal bodies there is insecurity of tenure.

It is most urgently necessary also to form a service of women civil assistant surgeons and sub-assistant surgeons or some such corresponding grades; eventually these should form the bulk of the medical women in the country. In several medical schools, especially in Bengal and the United Provinces, women sub-assistant surgeons are being trained, but the entire scheme for the creation of this class is still in its incipient stage.

At present there are no Government appointments for women doctors; there are a limited number of posts in the larger provincial hospitals and under municipal bodies, and in special Zenana hospitals. Women and children's hospitals are required in a considerable number of the larger towns; and these institutions should be provided with a staff of women doctors and women sub-assistant surgeons or subordinates. Staffing women's hospitals with women doctors is one of the most speedy ways of popularising Western medicine. Miss K. A. Platt, M.D., B.S., of the Lady Dufferin Women's Medical

Service, and Principal of the Lady Hardinge Medical College, Delhi, states: "As the result of ten years' work amongst both European and Indian women and children in various parts of India, I feel sure that the establishment of some civil medical service in which women are included is necessary." Personally I consider that these women doctors could be employed to attend the sick women and children of our Indian soldiers, when Indian Station Hospitals are provided with suitable accommodation for the purpose.

Were the present Women's Medical Service expanded and the conditions of that service improved it could undoubtedly be made the beginning of a movement for bringing the medical relief afforded by women doctors within the reach of the civil population. Assuming that such expansion will take place it should have, as part of its organization, a senior administrative woman doctor with the D.G., I.M.S., and a deputy in each province working in the office of the Surgeon-General or I.G.C.H. The qualifications of the women now working in India are such as to fit them for such work. Recruitment would be best effected by open competition; and Indian women should be equally eligible with Europeans. It is very desirable that successful candidates go through a course of tropical medicine in the School of Tropical Medicine in Calcutta before taking up their duties systematically; then work in one of the special women and children's hospitals or in the women and children's department of a civil general hospital for at least six months before being drafted to the towns and districts.

It is absolutely necessary that all women's hospitals should be regularly inspected and supervised as all the general and district hospitals are. This would be carried out by the I.G.C.H., and the provincial head of the women doctors, but such supervision does not receive much attention at present. It is important also that there should be a system of post-graduate training for women doctors in India. The general experience seems to be that women doctors, after five years' work in India, either stagnate or retrogress professionally unless they get the fillip of a post-graduate course. When systematic post-graduate courses are part of the routine medical education of the country, women doctors should take advantage of them.

If a Women's Medical Service were organized on sound lines for the whole country, with acceptable conditions, and a guaranteed security of tenure, it is possible that it would attract women doctors from the United Kingdom ; the pay and prospects of the present Women's Medical Service are not good enough to attract the best doctors. Many of us doubt whether the time has yet arrived for the creation of an Imperial Women's Medical Service in India. The existing prospects and conditions of life of women doctors as independent private practitioners in India are not sufficiently alluring, and comparatively few will venture to come to India from the United Kingdom in the present unstable state of indigenous political opinion and antagonism to British administration.

A " Junior Branch of the Women's Medical Service for India " has recently been created. It is included in the National Association for supplying female medical aid to the women of India, and is directed and controlled under the rules published by the Central Committee of that Association. Recruiting is carried out by the Central Committee, which includes the D.G., I.M.S., and the Honorary and Joint Secretaries of the Central Committee. There is a sub-committee which examines candidates as to their physical fitness, and gives permission to return to duty after periods of invaliding ; it may delegate its powers to local boards. The candidate for this service must be a British-born subject resident in India, possess a medical qualification registrable in the United Kingdom and in India, be between 24 and 30 years of age, unmarried or a widow, and present a certificate of health and moral character. Women of exceptional ability are enrolled under special conditions. The Central Committee appoints recruits to the various provinces. The candidates must engage for general service anywhere in India or Burma, and undergo a probationary period of one year, at the end of which time they are permanently appointed or their service terminated by order of the Central Committee on receipt of a report of the Provincial Committee of the Countess of Dufferin Fund. After confirmation service terminates at any time with three months' notice on either side; the Central Committee has power to dispense with the services of members at any time on paying three months' salary.

2. Training of Midwives

One of the saddest incidents in India is the death of thousands of women directly or indirectly from child-bearing, which arises chiefly from the unsatisfactory way in which their accouchements are conducted. This ceaseless tragedy is remediable, but if the eyes of the people are not opened to the appalling nature of this terrible death-toll, one apprehends that it will be some generations before any serious change for the better is brought about. In 1893–4, I gave the details of many cases of puerperal septicæmia that occurred in women I came across in practice during a few years—in several groups of cases the same *dhai* or native midwife was responsible for a succession of infections. One could also recite numerous instances illustrating the extraordinary barbarity connected with some of the methods adopted in difficult labour; these things are still going on—thousands of lives, mothers and infants, are lost because they have not efficient doctors and midwives to look after them during the lying-in period.

Parturient women in India are gravely neglected, especially among the poorer classes. Very often the lying-in room consists of a dirty, dark, ill-ventilated chamber, which in villages may be shared by cows or other animals, or these latter may occupy a shed or verandah conterminous with the chamber. Many are looked after by *dhais*, or quack midwives, who know nothing about hygiene or cleanliness in the accoucheur's sense; the result is often sepsis in the mother or tetanus in the child. For a period of ten years I was engaged in endeavouring to combat the tragic results of the deeds of these women, who are ignorant of the rudiments of cleanliness and have customs that cause puerperal septic infection in many of their cases. When in professional difficulties they sometimes leave their unfortunate victims, often after inflicting serious if not fatal injury.

Is there no method by which poor women can be provided with skilled aid during parturition at their own house or hut? Is there no means of ensuring that poor women can obtain the services of trained and reliable midwives for ordinary labour, to say nothing of help of a higher standard in difficult labour or in conditions associated with danger to the mother and child? The after-care of the health of mother and child also requires attention, for upon that depends the recuperation of the mother, fitting her to nurse her offspring, and the development and rearing of the child itself. The factors here are chiefly hygienic—pure air, proper feeding of the child, washing of clothes, etc. Too early undertaking of household duties and even labour in the field, and want of proper food often affect the mother's health. Here health visitors could do much by instruction in the proper way to nurse and feed babies and to treat the minor maladies to which babies are subject.

With the view of ameliorating these causes Lady Curzon, in 1903, started the Victoria Memorial Scholarship Fund; the money collected was to be utilized in the proper training of the *dhai*, or indigenous midwife class, whose calling is hereditary. The collection amounted to about £45,000, yielding £2,250 a year. This movement did not thrive, as the form of training given was altogether too theoretical; a large number of the midwives were old women, some were deaf or blind, and many of them started with the conviction that they had nothing to learn. In a report on this Fund it has recently been stated: "Improvement of the conditions of childbirth in India is a problem at least as difficult and at least as important as the prevention of plague, and it is only by patient work, frequently unsuccessful, and experiments constantly repeated, that a successful issue can be expected. In time to come the thanks of India will no doubt be given to those who have shown by practical experiment that supervision of hereditary *dhais* is not only desirable but possible. In this connection the Committee would particularly mention the names of Miss Hewlett, of Amritsur, Dr. Agnes Henderson, of Nagpur, Dr. Gertrude Stuart, of Quetta, and Dr. Maud Allen, as deserving the gratitude of the women of India. As regards the class of women to be trained, the Committee feels the warmest interest in all efforts to train and assist midwives of a superior class, but it feels that until proof is given that the majority of women in the provinces, rich and poor alike, are employing these midwives for natural labour, the funds of the Victoria Memorial Scholarship must be expended entirely for the improvement of the hereditary *dhai* class."

The object of this Fund was to train indigenous midwives in the female wards of hospitals and in female training schools so as to enable them to carry on their hereditary calling in harmony with the religious feelings of the people and gradually improve their traditional methods in the light of modern sanitation and medical knowledge; to grant scholarships varying according to place and circumstances; and to send, when desirable, qualified female teachers who understood the vernacular to outlying districts and posts for the benefit of midwives attending a course of elementary instruction, funds for the above purpose to be granted as far as possible according to the interest received on the sums raised in each locality.

A question that has been a source of much anxiety and thought in India is whether the work of improving the hereditary *dhai* class should be continued, or whether efforts in this direction should be abandoned and replaced by endeavours to create a better class of midwife. Opinions are divided. Several civil administrative medical officers, civil surgeons and others consider that the latter is the best solution. On the other hand the majority of women doctors who have devoted much time to the question declare it to be impossible as a practical measure, notwithstanding its soundness in theory. "It is true the hereditary *dhai* class are unwilling to be taught, make unsatisfactory pupils, and often after training are no better than before, while women of the other classes are obedient and amenable, may have some education, and absorb new ideas readily. On the other hand it is stated that it is impossible at present to get a sufficient number of educated Indian women to replace indigenous *dhais*. It may be possible in the capital cities (excellent work in this direction is now being done in Calcutta, Bombay and Madras) but it is not possible throughout the districts of India, where the population is scattered over wide areas and where women are being sought in vain to take up posts as compounders, nurses, teachers, etc. Next it is argued that a woman of higher class expects a fee much larger than the middle and lower class Indian family is as a rule prepared to give, or able to afford. She is also unwilling to do all the work in the home the hereditary *dhai* is expected to do, and this forms a very practical obstacle to her employment in poor families. In many cases trained midwives have been retained by municipalities and it has been found that they have attended few cases of natural labour, even after years of work, and this even though the people were quite ready to look upon them as doctors and call them in for abnormal cases." One can vouch for the accuracy of this statement as regards our cantonment hospitals in India, in many of which we have *dhais* and arrangements for lying-in cases that are seldom used by the people for whom they are intended. "Some claim that the hereditary *dhai* when young is found to be adaptable, intelligent, willing, with a certain hereditary instinct for her work, which, other things being equal, makes her a better pupil than the women of other classes."

The opinion of most women doctors therefore is "that for general improvement of child-birth in India work among hereditary *dhais* must be continued, but that it is useless unless it is combined with some scheme of supervision of their work by means of midwife supervisors."

The best solution to this very difficult problem has still to be worked out, and its importance shows that it should be studied and experimented on by provincial governments, civil administrative medical officers, civil surgeons, medical women, better class midwives, and women of the educated classes in India, all of whom should make suggestions for improving the conditions. In some places it will be found that satisfactory progress can be made, in others that improvement of conditions is either impracticable or so extremely difficult as to be insurmountable. I am disposed to think that much help could be rendered both by the Imperial and Provincial Governments in the amelioration of the dreadful conditions referred to and the suffering and the deplorable loss of life greatly reduced. Under the most favourable circumstances it will take many years to achieve success.

So far practically all effort to mitigate the lot of parturient women in India has emanated from Europeans, men and women, especially from women doctors, who are brought intimately into contact with the existing conditions. It is difficult for people brought up in Western views to understand how the better class educated Indians can know that this sad tragedy is going on around them from one year's end to another, without being roused to remove, or, at least, to ameliorate it; that it can be greatly alleviated by a sustained, widespread and well-organized effort patiently carried out, I entertain no doubt whatever.

Assuming that miracles cannot be wrought in this matter, it does not seem "humanly possible to replace the thousands of these indigenous *dhais* that carry on their work throughout the country. Is it not possible, however, to absorb them into a large scheme and gradually train them in elementary midwifery and the care of infants?

9

They might be induced to attend demonstrations and lectures at definite centres. Even in this there are difficulties; many of these women are totally illiterate and some of those who can read and write the vernaculars are so imbued with prejudice against our methods that the task of teaching them is not light. A further obstacle is that many mothers themselves are not in sympathy with Western methods, preferring to follow the practices of their ancestors. The whole question bristles with difficulties; I can offer no solution, and I much doubt if anyone else can.

3. Infant Mortality

Another melancholy and perpetual experience is the high infant mortality and the unfortunate conditions of child-life in India. This has aroused much sympathy and been the subject of many philanthropic efforts, the most stable of which has been the organization associated with the name of Lady Dufferin. That benevolent and noble woman made the first fruitful attempt to provide lady doctors for India.

The present lamentable position of child welfare in India is shown by the appalling death-rate of infants in some of the chief cities. The death-rate in Calcutta in 1912 was 259 per 1,000 registered births, and in the four years 1895, 1900, 1901, and 1902 it exceeded 400 per 1,000, that of Nagpur (C.P.) in 1912 was 420·6, in 1915 it was 312, and in 1916 it was 310; for Bombay in 1914 it was 325, in 1915 329, and in 1916 it reached 387 per 1,000 births. In rural areas where the conditions of infant life are worse, in many places it is higher. In general terms it may be said that in late years in India the birth-rate has been falling and the death-rate of infants rising. This heavy toll of infant life arises from numerous causes, among which may be mentioned—the dreadful conditions under which parturition is conducted, immaturity and ignorance of the mothers, defective feeding, and insanitary environment. According to a recent report of the Health Officer of Calcutta, 94 per 1,000 of the infant deaths occur during the first week of life, and arise from a want of knowledge on the part of the mother, premature birth, debility, neglect and "nine-day tetanus." The startling figures regarding Calcutta initiated the laudable movement of providing trained midwives to conduct accouchements among the poorer classes, women and health visitors to advise prospective mothers regarding the hygiene of pregnancy and the rearing of infants. The effect of this movement was to reduce the infant death-rate very considerably. Similar praiseworthy schemes are being carried out in Madras and Bombay, and in a few other capital cities of provinces.

Any plan of improvement should include protection of the woman during pregnancy, the infant and the child. The health of the mother is undermined by early and repeated pregnancy, prolonged lactation, poor food, overwork and, in many cases, malarial infection more or less chronic. The health of the mother affects the future health and vitality of the infant. A complete scheme would afford protection before birth, during birth and afterwards. Still-births and death from immaturity are common; miscarriages are very frequent, and in many cases become a perverted habit. Among the more common serious diseases in mothers before parturition are—abortions, anæmia, malaria, and convulsions, all of which could be treated during pregnancy; sepsis, a preventable disease, is common. If all women were under skilled care and advice during pregnancy it is probable that a considerable percentage of still-births, abortions, etc., would be prevented. The ideal way would be to get mothers to attend courses of instruction, and health visitors to advise them during pregnancy at their houses; the effect would be maintenance of the health of the mothers, and this would do the same for the child.

INDEX